Mother, Do Not Weep for Me

Published by Morning Light Press 2010
Copyright © 2010 by Morning Light Press

ISBN: 978-1-59675-034-0

Cover Image: © Ben Koralek
Image of Ben Koralek: ©Shape East, Cambridge, UK

Printed on acid-free, recycled paper in Canada.

Library of Congress Cataloging-in-Publication Data
Koralek, Jenny.
 Mother, do not weep for me : a son's life remembered with joy / Jenny Koralek.
   p. cm.
 ISBN 978-1-59675-034-0 (alk. paper)
 1. Koralek, Ben, 1967-2006. 2. Koralek, Ben, 1967-2006--Death and burial. 3.
Koralek, Jenny. 4. Mothers and sons--England. 5. Sons--England--Biography. 6.
Chronically ill--England--Biography. 7. Sons--Death. 8. Premature death. 9. Parental
grief. 10. Women authors, English--Biography I. Title.
 CT788.K67K67 2010
 306.874'3--dc22
 [B]
                                2009050467

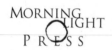

10881 North Boyer Road, Sandpoint, ID 83864   morninglightpress.com

Mother, Do Not Weep for Me

A Son's Life Remembered with Joy

Jenny Koralek

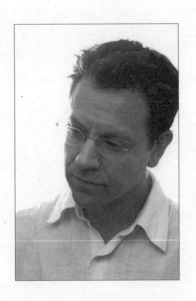

Death Announcement

KORALEK, Ben (Benjamin Paul), aged 39, on 6 July 2006 suddenly and unexpectedly, in Addenbrooke's Hospital, Cambridge. Adored, adoring and tender husband and father of his "lovely girls," Vicky Anning Koralek and Jenna Grace (22 months). Most beloved son of Paul and Jenny Koralek; dearest brother of Katy Ricks and Lucy Williams, very dear uncle of Lilly and Jake and truly loved by his brothers-in-law, David Ricks and Luke Williams. Life-loving, courageous and gracious, he could not have been more loved by all who knew him . . .

—from *The Times*, Thursday 13 July 2006

Cause

Conclusion of the post mortem report:

On balance the changes in the heart are of a myopathic process of uncertain aetiology but may be related to his underlying ulcerative colitis. The changes would be sufficient to account for death at this time.

The cause of death should therefore read:

1a. Cardiomyopathy of uncertain cause. 2. Ulcerative colitis.

With respect to Ben's heart not only did he have the marked dilation prone to generate bad rhythms and arrest, but also other contributors of sudden death emerge from the report including abnormal thickness of muscle; inflammation from chemo and/or virus infection. (Ben's resistance was lowered by ulcerative colitis and chemo); the inflammation of heart muscle seen was similar to instances known in ulcerative colitis; electrolyte imbalance; these and several other factors combined and interacted to generate a fatal heart rhythm or stop the heart.

I don't think one can isolate a single cause of Ben's cardiac arrest. The causes were multiple and interacted.

> —Comments and explanations from Distinguished Professor of Cardiology, Dr. Richard S. Crampton, University of Virginia, on the post mortem report from Papworth Hospital, Cambridge.

Preface

I wish to make it clear that this memoir has been written entirely from my particular perspective of what happened to my son, having absolutely no right to try at second remove to describe what other members of the family experienced or are experiencing.

Any understanding, any capacity that I may have to stand under this suffering, I owe entirely to my direct experience for over fifty years of the teaching of G. I. Gurdjieff, and the very great help received during all those years from many of his pupils, particularly Henri and Nano Tracol, Louise and William J. Welch, Lise Zuber and Bernard Courtenay-Mayers, all of whom watched lovingly over Ben during his childhood and early adult life.

It is not important how long one lives, but whether one develops something which can give meaning to life.

—Jeanne de Salzmann

Now, you are mother. Do you understand?

—Olga de Hartmann, 1966

Vapor is Ever Rising

This grand show is eternal. It is always sunrise somewhere: the dew is never all dried up at once: a shower is forever falling, vapor is ever rising. Eternal sunrise, eternal sunset, eternal dawn and gloaming, on sea and continents and islands, each in its turn, as the round earth rolls.

—John Muir

So much of what I am now experiencing of this Pacific coast, this great West of the mythical USA has come to me from generosity, the giving of others, the Giving of the Season of Summer, the giving of the Sun, family, colleagues, beloved friends, strangers; all with a generosity of Spirit, and I have found that my spirit has responded. I am grateful regularly and frequently and it makes me more relaxed, more stretched, perhaps even more "spacious" (as Sogyal Rinpoche[1] would say) . . . and as I write this, watching pelicans fishing amidst the crashing waves of the East Pacific, something strikes me with the pounding thunder of the Ocean's white and grey waters: perhaps I could maintain the attitude of foreigner/traveler and not know the answers while remaining in the state of Gratitude: I would like to try . . . for living as a child of these two stars ("Not-Knowing-Answers" and "Gratitude"

---

1 Tibetan Buddhist teacher and founder of the RIGPA centers, author of *The Tibetan Book of Living and Dying.*

has made me very happy and contented and I'm sure a more human Human being.

—Ben Koralek, Rialto Beach, Washington, August, 1997

Table of Contents

Chapter 1

Mother, Do Not Weep for Me

Thursday 6 July—8:00 p.m.: "Hullo Mum, Ben here. Running out of credit on my phone . . . I'll call you back, or you call me . . . "

Thursday 6 July—8:30 p.m.: "Hullo Mum, bit of a bummer they want me to stay in for two more weeks to treat the fungal lesions with IV antibiotics . . . Can you sort things to help Vicky with visiting etc.? She's finding all this very hard . . . take care of her . . . she's the center of my life . . . Speak to you tomorrow, Mum."

My son is dead. My son is dead.

The little black phone by my bed. Every night I look at it. Every night I can tell myself: Well, at least it will never ring again at two minutes past midnight and a voice say: "He's had another cardiac arrest"—a voice that had the wit not to tell me he is already dead.

———

"I trust you, Mum. Am I dying?" And I could honestly say, "No," but knowing that if he had been I would have had to say "Yes."

That was *last* year. *Last* July. After the *first* cardiac arrest.

And now I am the questioner: "Is he dead?" I ask his father. He nods. It is now three minutes into 7 July 2006. He is on the little black phone to the duty doctor at the hospital. We are sitting side by side on the edge of the bed, the bed where we have lain for 43 years, in the very room, the very space within which I gave birth to him (8 lbs. 12

oz. and masses of blonde hair) on 14 June 1967 at 10:15 in the morning—a hot bright blue June morning, in the room where I would feed him, sitting in an old bentwood chair from the Vienna of his paternal grandparents . . .

What happens if you die from one second to the next?

"Unprepared?"

Angels must then come.

We didn't pause after we heard. We didn't stop and sit down and be with him.

Did our shock, our weeping and pain distress him? Hinder him? Add to his own shock?

Did he know he was going to die soon?

Did he have an almost unconscious premonition if that isn't a contradiction in terms?

"He's had another cardiac arrest," says the voice, the calm voice of his mother-in-law up in York. "We are getting in the car now and going straight down to Cambridge. Someone will go with Vicky to the hospital . . . A good friend . . . " I think that's what she says . . .

"Is he dead?" I ask again.

His father nods again.

A few more words with the doctor.

Hangs up.

"They found him too late. Collapsed in the shower. Thought he'd been there about twenty minutes before he was discovered. They did everything they could, but it was too late."

We sit side by side. Not touching. But looking into each other's eyes. Stunned. Speechless. Total shock. Every banal adjective anyone cares to offer.

Then at some point I say: "We must tell the girls."

I phone Lucy. Phone rings and rings. I remember they don't have a phone in their bedroom. They can't hear it ringing. Remember Lilly has a mobile which I have often teased her for never turning it off. Search frantically in my bag for crumpled postcard covered with family mobile numbers along with myriad hospital numbers for all the wards he has been in over the past eighteen months. Find Lil's number. Dial. She answers immediately, poor girl, expecting some insomniac friend. It must by then have been 12:30. I ask her to get Mum. She obviously can hear something is terribly wrong.

Half starts to ask. But I just ask her again to go and get Lucy. She does. Lucy comes to the phone. I tell her. She bursts into tears. I don't remember what we said to each other, but eventually we hang up.

Phone Katy. Same thing. No response. Remember they don't have a phone upstairs either. Hang up in despair. Almost at once she rings. "Mum? Did you ring just now?" I tell her yes and why. She weeps. David is there. He is comforting her, she says. We agree to talk in morning.

Lucy rings. They are coming over now. They arrive somewhere between 1:30 and 2 a.m., speechless, numb; children sleepy and silent. They crash in my study. Jake dives onto bed and under duvet; Lil uncomfortably on makeshift bed on floor. I think we others had some tea. We all go to bed, but before long I am up again and go into the garden. It is a warm summer's night. It is now 7 July and Ben is dead.

My son is dead.

My son is dead.

I rock backwards and forwards while upstairs Paul sleeps; everyone else sleeps, or do they? Not much, Lucy and Luke tell me next day.

What do I remember next?

Getting read to go to Cambridge, to Addenbrooke's to see him in the chapel.

Not room for us all in minicab. Jake goes with his mother to find a taxi. We meet at King's Cross. They all buy Cornish pasties. How can they *eat*?

We find Katy and David at hospital. Long wait. At last, escorted by kind woman down into bowels of hospital into the little waiting room, the little room where he lies.

Paul, Lucy, Katy and I go in.

He lies there so lovely still. A big bruise. The left hand corner of his mouth still curved in a small smile. I kiss his icy forehead. Others lean over. Others kiss him.

We stand and stand and stand there looking looking looking.
Luke and David have joined us and I think then Lilly. And then—Jake, who had sworn he wouldn't come in. Would NOT come in. But he does . . . Stands by Ben's head . . .

We stand and stand and stand.

I kiss him again and again and murmur, "Love. Love. Love. Light. Light. Light."
Some go out. We go out. But go back a few last times. A last few kisses and, "Love, love, love, darling. Light. Light. Light."

We go back to Ben and Vicky's house. Katy drives us. On the way I remember a message that several of our close friends will meet at 4 p.m. to "think" of us—once we would have dared say "pray" for us. I look at my watch. It is 4 p.m. I nudge Paul and point at my watch. He takes my hand.

Vicky all in black. We hug silently. Her mother is there. She embraces me so kindly. "I'm so sorry. I'm so sorry." I know she really loved him.
I hear Lucy say to Vicky: "The last thing he said to me on the phone was 'Vicky is the center of my life.'"

Little Jenna runs about from one to another of us, almost as if saying: *No, you are not the one, you are not the one.* She is 22 months old. She has been told, as she so often was, that Daddy is with the "doc-docs." But she doesn't seem to be unhappy. Luke and Jake go out into the garden and play with her. The girls sit close to V. Three lovely women. Katy's and Lucy's voices a low murmur of concern and sympathy . . .

I think we drink tea and are offered cake. Don't remember drinking or eating.

I say to Jake, "It is noble of you, darling, to play with Jenna." He says, "Well, she's very good at cheering you up."

Katy and David take us to the station.

I remember nothing about getting home. I remember nothing about crying.

Next day a very good friend calls from France in the middle of rehearsing a play for a festival.

"Dear Jenny," he says, "I have always sensed that you were with him *all the way*."

"I don't understand anything," I tell him. "Whatever I thought I understood, now I don't. What the hell do we all think we are *doing* with our lives?" "That is *the* question," he says. "The one we need to ask every single day . . . "

And as I write I suddenly remember an earlier conversation with him last year, not long after Ben's recovery from his cardiac arrest and just before he was about to start on his chemotherapy. It was a serious exchange about death, when he reminded me that all sacred traditions lay enormous stress on the need for life to be understood as a preparation for death.

I tell Paul that same day that I would like to go and sit quietly with some wise friends. I phone. They say: "Yes, of course. Come." And Lucy? And her husband? "But of course."

We go to their house. Their daughter is there who has endured from birth many difficulties with her body. "I have often wanted to tell you," I say to her, "how much in common you have with Ben, maybe because you both have had to suffer so much; I think that is why you both have such immense feeling for others—compassion, one could say."

"And I often wanted to say that to you," she replied, "about Ben." She smiles tenderly.

We sit in a circle in their sitting room. We sit unmoving and profoundly silent for about half an hour.

My form dissolves . . . cells, tissues, the all of it. Concomitant with this dissolution an increase in a sense of my own melting of too, too solid flesh . . . And I meet him in formlessness. Sense that this is the one and only way to be with him—in consciousness. Now I weep quietly.

But later with outrage, refusal, disbelief.

NO NO NO NO NO NO NO NO NO NO NO NO NO NO NO

I can't bear it.

—

Every day between his death and the funeral the sun shone. It was extremely hot. Butterflies everywhere and birdsong strong. Hugely aware of nature. Quality of attention very fine—never known such quality before. Must be from the shock, shocking me into life. Tingling with life. Before and after the funeral, feelings very open indeed to everyone, loving, caring for needs of all kinds—very good home-cooked food, fresh linen for guests, flowers in bedrooms, hangers for clothes, boxes of tissues. Soup. And accompanied by very vivid memories of the past, things from my childhood, my parents and family springing up, almost at times such great chunks of my life flashing past I wonder if it is akin to what has been described happens to the drowning; after all what is happening is for me a kind of drowning, a kind of dying . . . Does there *have* to be a shock of such power before one can awaken? Can it be sustained? I felt it diminish and drain away during following months.

—

"There is another kind of time." I hear again, after more than twenty years, the voice of Henri Tracol, speaking to Paul who had just heard that his father had died.

"Dear Jenny, you were with him every step of the way." I return to these words, too, often.

—

I long for a visitation, a dream vision; but they do not come.

—

What is the taste, the feel of grief?

A lead weight in solar plexus. A ghastly fluttering like a million butterflies. A tingling all through body.

Then knowing weeping is coming. Other times little yelps. And rocking, rocking of the body in bed, or for many many days between 5 and 6 a.m. out in the garden at Cottage in the already heating up day, rocking rocking back and forth on a bench or the concrete ledge of studio . . . rocking rocking. Hollow tapping of teeth . . .

———

Where are you, darling?

———

A butterfly came to Lucy and me on the terrace in the already baking morning heat, breakfasting alone a few days before the funeral; a butterfly came and settled on the empty chair between us and stayed there for an hour, opening and closing its jewel wings, as, like a drowning woman, I clung to the spiritual help I had long ago received from Henri Tracol[1] and William Segal[2], and was now sharing with my daughter.

A butterfly circled the flower-covered grave the day after the funeral, when Paul and I went down there to try and absorb the truth of it.

———

It is over. He is not in that shower room any more. He is not sick from the chemo anymore. His mouth doesn't hurt anymore. There are no tubes, no pumps in him. It is over—for him. It is I who return there. He doesn't. He is free, free of the physical and mental and emotional suffering. F R E E.

---

1 "I pray for help, I pray for help: I know it is there for sure."
2 "I can be infinitely more relaxed than I am. I can have infinitely more sensation; I can be breathed; I can receive a thought from Above."

———

His heart has been taken to Papworth Hospital . . .

Vicky talks to them:

It will take at least four weeks—maybe more to complete the post mortem so do you want to postpone the funeral?

No.

Would you like us to dispose of the heart after the post mortem?

No.

Would you like us to keep the heart for research purposes which would only ever be conducted at Papworth?

No—we want the heart back to be buried in his grave.

———

There was talk in the corridor outside the ITU of a defibrillator.

There was talk of putting him into an induced arrest to see—what?

Twice he went to Papworth.

It was decided not to do that test. Why? Too dangerous?

———

Ellen directs me to the NASA website and a spectacular photo of a heart-shaped nebula—somehow consoling to see this shape appear cosmically . . . myriad "stars" sparkling, glittering . . .

———

What helps?

One thought that helps: In the words of Hui Neng, the Sixth Patriarch in the Zen tradition, he has found again his "original face, the face he had before he was born."

———

Dark thoughts—imaginings, unanswered questions . . .

What have they done to him to arrive at the post mortem conclusions?

How long does it take for a body to decompose?

Does our grief, his grief, hinder him?

Where is he?

Is he in the bardos of the Tibetans Buddhists? In the gaps they say we must pass through before being "born again"? Or has he gone immediately in light, to light?

I decide to "read" to him the "instructions" from what we all call *The Tibetan Book of the Dead*, but which they call *The Great Liberation on Hearing*. Or at least to murmur daily and often, "stay with the bright clear lights, darling; not the dull ones which will pull you back down again but the bright ones . . . guiding you to a Pure Land . . . "

———

Sometimes, particularly on a "bad" day, I become aware of my voice, an automaton, a robotic voice, or my talking as if it was coming from someone else, a feeling of being completely hollow, an empty shell, from which the snail life has vanished, been consumed. Disintegrated. Diminished. Not Jenny any more. Not there any more.

I catch glimpse of self in a mirror . . . who is that woman? Is that me?

———

A dry, harsh grief has set in. I weep less, but great pangs overwhelm me: I might suddenly weep forever, but I mustn't. Not at bedtime. The two worst times are then—bedtime and in middle of the afternoon, God knows why then. I understand the bed time—I see that bloody little black phone . . . The day is over, distractions are over . . . I start to want Ben to "appear" to me when I sleep . . . When it's bad and so as not to disturb Paul, I get up again and wander about . . .

Chapter 2

Day of Funeral

What do I remember of that day, 19 July 2006?

It was extremely hot—about 90 F, no clouds.

Regardless of the great heat I made soup—specially for Vicky as I felt that might be, as for me, about all she could get down.

I think we were all a bit "hyper," running on this strange energy which seemed to have kicked in very soon after Ben died. I continued to be aware of a very high degree of attention, fine, sensitive, "une attention azimuth"[1] as Henri Tracol would have called it—able to take in everything around me—nature, people, needs, priorities.

Everyone was busy with something.

At some point in that long morning we went to look at the grave. I felt I had to look at it—at the deep, deep hole. Had to face that *before* the burial later in the afternoon.

We took iced water for the gravedigger, a genial character, Yorick, came to mind. We told him—no, I told him, that he was digging our son's grave, that he was only 39.

Quietly indignant, "The good ones always go young, never seems to be the layabouts."

---

1 An Arabic mathematical term: "the arc of the horizon between the meridian of a place and a vertical circle passing through any celestial body."

We put out lots of food for lunch for people to have, or not have, when they wanted it.

I have a memory of showers being taken, a general flurry, but a quiet one, of preparation.

The young caterers coming...

I remember my sister, limping from a bad knee, coming toward me in the garden, her lovely son hugging me, incoherent tender sounds of love, her lovely daughter embracing Lucy and their weeping.

We drove ourselves to the church; Vicky and her family followed the hearse from the funeral directors.

I remember walking toward the church alone, while Paul parked the car.

I remember an old, old friend in the shade of the trees coming forward weeping to embrace me.

I remember a beloved cousin in tears at the back of the church coming to me, murmuring "darling" and hugging me.

I remember watching four young men carrying in the willow coffin: two were Ben's brothers-in-law; one his best man at his wedding; one a friend since childhood who bowed to the coffin as they laid it gently down.

I remember reading the poem, *The Noble Nature*[1], by Ben Jonson, with Ben's godfather on my left and another Ben, "son," I said, "of our Ben's late godmother..."

---

1 It is not growing like a tree
    In bulk, doth make man better be;
    Or standing long an oak, three hundred year,
    To fall a log at last, dry, bald, and sere:
    A lily of a day
    Is fairer far in May,
    Although it fall and die that night
    It was the plant and flower of Light.
    In small proportions we just beauties see;
    And in short measures life may perfect be.

I remember, when I came to the words *plant and flower of Light*, turning toward the coffin . . .

I remember our daughters reading . . .

I remember running across the aisle to hold Vicky's hand when her mother went up to the lectern to read.

I remember Paul speaking . . .

I remember Canon Hulbert speaking about Ben at some worthwhile length, almost as if he had known him well, this thanks to his immense generosity in coming to talk to us all three times in the days before . . . .

I remember him praying for Ben and for us all, naming each one of us in turn, not forgetting a single person . . .

I remember following the coffin out of the church . . .

I remember Vicky kissing the coffin before they took it from the hearse and heard myself say out loud to no-one in particular, *I would like to have done that*, and hearing to my horror shades of my mother, ego in the voice, *me, me, me,* which pulled me up, remembering again must always take second place, third place, fourth place. Vicky first.

I remember standing at the graveside with Paul on my right.

I don't remember who was on my left.

Was it Lucy? Yes, I think it was Lucy.

I think each of us at that point was completely, utterly alone, in a great terrible solitude, unable to help anyone else, yet holding hands . . .

I remember letting out a cry as the coffin was lowered, *Oh, darling* . . .

And feeling a warm hand on my shoulder . . . someone standing behind me . . .

I knew it was my son-in-law, Luke, Lucy's husband . . . and was grateful.

I remember as we turned to leave noticing a young good-looking man standing apart from everyone, tall, jet black thick straight hair, still with the same gentle dimpled smile I remembered from his childhood . . . and realized it was Ben's very first friend, Tom. When they were introduced, aged 4, they dived under the tea table and didn't come out till it was time to go home. A little while later they went to the same school, endured the same bullying, and in our back garden reveled in messy games involving melting down their toy cars into interesting sculpture, falling about at jokes only they understood and only they thought were funny, and until discovered by their mothers, cruelly crushing snails against a wall. When they were six, I took them to see *Peter Pan*; they were so entranced, dumbstruck, enchanted that I can still hear their seats banging up or down so little were they able to stay seated for more than a minute at a time throughout the whole performance. And now, 35 years on, here was Tom standing in a Sussex churchyard saying good-bye to *his* first friend about whom he had written: "My friendship with Ben was one of the first and greatest in my life. It really showed me what a wonderful, hilarious, fun thing friendship can be . . . "

A year after Ben's death I was to find Ben's 9-year old account of their initial friendship in his *My Backward Autobiography*:

I can remember when Mum and Dad said, "Come on Ben, come and see your new school." But I said, "No." When I was at that school I came home with brused [sic] legs, knees and arms. I was always being bashed up by older children. That was the bad side of it but the good side of it was that I met my best friend there . . . I remember when we had a fire drill and the headmistress said, "You were not ready," me and Tom said, "BREK," so it came out as "You are not REDY BREK . . . [1]"

---

1 The brand name of a rather disgusting pre-cooked porridge. A year later I also found this poem Ben wrote when he was about 12, describing the bullying he and Tom experienced, and already showing signs of his adult concern about what education and its environment should not be:

The Walls That Swayed
Children running, shouting, playing,
Innocently blind to other people.
Separate games and groups of boys and girls
Enjoying "free time."

I remember thanking the funeral director.

And then at the tea back at the house, the young ones all sitting up on the lawn, the old ones down by the house.

I didn't want to talk to anyone but people came up and said things . . . I found the grandchildren and their best friends in a huddle at the back of the house away from people . . .

Restlessly I wandered here and there . . . carried Jenna Grace up to the paddling pool . . .

Then . . . all is a blank.

But later—that day?—Lucy suggested that it was as if great love was pouring down on all of us. And I wondered, and still wonder, whether that was so to speak Ben's love for us all pouring down on us, telling us that all was well with him?

Free time that was enjoyed by all, behind bars!
High fences planted in concrete,
In front of high walls with windows and red bricks.
Dividing the fences and walls were
Floors of concrete, and a scarce square of grass
With a pole of wood protruding from its base.

Two boys stood pinned to wall,
On a bench or a strip of wood.
"If you don't bring me and me mate 5p each me
Dad'll kill you!" ordered an enforcer.
I, terrified, agreed to this plan along with my friend
And they left us like statues.
Slowly we walked away and turned
To see the walls sway,
With tallness, oldness and thinness,
As if shaking with disapproval.

Chapter 3

The Heart

Very soon after the funeral I began to fret about his heart.

For a while there was wild talk about how to transport it from Papworth Hospital to us in Sussex: A white van to be found through the Yellow Pages? Someone's cousin's van?

Vicky to bring it with her in the car (among the toddler gear and the luggage)? How would she endure that and, for that matter, Ben's sister, Lucy, too who would be there as she would be going to help Vicky with the journey?

Eventually, in great distress, I called a very dear, lifelong friend, an Episcopalian Minister and—like the Canon who conducted the funeral—a very exceptional man of the cloth.

"Jenny," he said in his strong, warm Virginian voice, "Ben had a noble heart.

"Did you know that in the olden days when a king of France died his heart was always removed and laid to rest in the cathedral of St Denis?

"Did you know that when Chopin died his heart was taken from Paris to Warsaw and buried in the Cathedral there?

"Whatever you decide to do, the heart should be treated royally with utmost respect."

Vicky asked advice from the Patient Liaison Officer at Papworth about what to do, how to proceed.

He said first and foremost we should be guided by our hearts and not our heads.

We could leave it to the Papworth Trust, where it would only be used for research there and never anywhere else.

She asked if it could be cremated so we could scatter the ashes onto the grave.

He said if it was incinerated there would be no ashes.

He said it could be returned to Addenbrooke's Hospital, correctly (vacuum) packed and that it was not necessary for police or funeral directors to transport it—we could do that if we wished.

In the end, clear and appropriate thinking prevailed and it was taken to the funeral directors who had arranged the funeral, a box chosen, and his name engraved on a little brass plate with a line from the lovely poem by C. Day-Lewis chosen by Vicky to go into the Order of Service.

And so on 18 August, a grey, damp cool day so very different from the fierce, relentless heat of the July days from his death until well after the funeral, we met at the Cottage where V. was staying with her closest friend, who had come all the way from New Zealand to spend some time with her.

Leaving Jenna Grace happy with her big cousins, we went to the nearby graveyard, the girls walking down carrying flowers.

We are met at the gate by the very young woman from the funeral directors', dressed for funereal hunting in a black coat, white shirt, long black skirt and a silken top hat.

She murmurs well intended noises of sympathy and something about "closure" . . .

Then mercifully the Canon arrives, embraces us, says nothing.

V. and I have gathered lots of flower petals from the garden. Katy carries two little stone pots containing lavender and rosemary.

The girl is holding the box with a hairy piece of twine tied round it. We stand at the foot of the grave which has been partially dug up revealing a deep narrow hole.

The Canon speaks sparingly of the possibility of growth through suffering.

He prays briefly, quoting St. Paul ("For I am persuaded that neither death, nor life, nor angels, nor principalities, nor powers, nor things present, nor things to come, Nor height, nor depth . . . shall be able to separate us from the love of God . . . ").

V. reads the C. Day-Lewis poem:
> His laughter was better than birds in the morning,
> his smile
> Turned the edge of the wind, his memory
> Disarms death and charms the surly grave.
> Early he went to bed, too early we
> Saw his light put out; yet we could not grieve
> More than a little while,
> For he lives in the earth around us, laughs from the sky.

Her friend reads a letter she has written to Ben recalling with love their twenty-year-long friendship and her gladness that he lies at rest in such a beautiful, peaceful place.

Canon Hulbert looks at the rest of us as if to say, *Do any of you wish to say something?*

I shake my head slightly.

The young funeral parlor girl walks along the line so that we can in turn each touch the little box.

V. scatters the flower petals into the grave . . .

The young girl slowly lowers the box by the twiny string . . .

V. comes forward carrying five red roses, *One for each year we were together*, and lays them on top of the box.

By now many of us are weeping silently.

I think Canon Hulbert blessed us.

We turn to one another and embrace one another.

And quietly, silently leave.

The gravedigger is sitting in his truck on the lane.

The same gravedigger who dug the grave initially . . .

We find the grandchildren quietly happy together.

We sit round the dining room table for a hearty lunch, swiftly prepared earlier by Vicky's capable friend.

Then Luke drives us to the station.

I remember nothing else about that day. Nothing.

Chapter 4

Decades of Illness

Every decade brought Ben a new, life-threatening illness.

But when exactly did it all begin?

Did it begin even when he was in the womb?

The year before he was born I became quite ill with hepatitis. When at last I was nearly better, the doctor surprised me by seriously counseling me on no account to get pregnant for at least 6 months to a year.

Three months later I discovered I was indeed pregnant, and was well until the 6th month when suddenly I developed an inflammation and infection of the gall bladder with high fever and much pain. Our GP arrived out of hours rather excitedly, and dramatically informed me that he had sent for a consultant gastroenterologist to come and examine me and advise what to do in order, if possible, to avoid surgery, which the baby would certainly not survive.

The great man duly arrived and decided instead that I should be treated with hefty doses of antibiotics for the remaining three months of the pregnancy.

The cholecystitis subsided and I went to full term without any problems. Ben weighed nearly 9 lbs at birth and until the age of 4 was a healthy, lively child.

When he was four years old he developed pneumococcal meningitis.

This was 1972. It is hard to believe now, when there is a much better understanding of the symptoms, that there was a terrible delay before a correct diagnosis was reached. He had recently recovered from mumps. But a few weeks later developed a large swollen gland on one side of his neck. He was clearly unwell, drooping about, lying on the sofa, or under a tree. We were down in the country at that point. I was sufficiently anxious to move him into our bedroom for the night, and heard him grinding his teeth, restless, but not yet feverish. By the time we got back to London he was clearly very unwell. Grizzly, complaining of a pain in his head, his neck. Suddenly he spiked a very high temperature, bouts of projectile vomiting began, an immense irritability, loss of appetite, dislike of light and every now and then, shrieking and if not shrieking, talking to me in a terrifyingly unrecognizable croaky voice. Of course we called our homeopathic doctor (we were going through a phase of "rejecting" orthodox medicine and were in the care of a charismatic homeopath, now long dead, of some fame at that time). He pronounced that Ben had a bad flu, and prescribed the remedy, bryonia. As he left I asked him could it be meningitis (and from that moment on always trusted a mother's diagnostic instinct). He was very angry with me. "Don't even think of that!" he thundered. "Do you *want* him to have it?"

Tossing and turning in his bed, visibly losing weight (his vertebrae becoming more and more defined), clearly very ill, I saw that he had developed a rash. I asked for a home visit from one of our NHS doctors, who said he had German measles. And left.

By the end of that long day Ben was delirious. The homeopath told me to bring him to his clinic where he would nurse him himself. Fool that I was, and watched by his terrified younger sister, I carried my struggling, screaming child into a mini-cab. To the driver's alarm I had the greatest difficulty in restraining Ben.

I took him to the homeopath who had him put to bed and began treating him with I know not what. I left my child lying there, calmer now, pale and completely unaware of anyone and went home, re-assured—I can hardly believe this, even now—that he was in good hands . . .

At about 5 a.m. the next morning we were awoken by a phone call from the homeopath telling me that he had himself admitted Ben to Great Ormond Street Hospital as he had become very worried by how ill he was and advised us to come there immediately. Within minutes of this call, we received another one from the sister on the ward at the hospital, almost ordering us to come *immediately*.

When we arrived we were not allowed into Ben's room, but through the glass we saw him thrashing about surrounded by gowned and masked doctors and nurses, battling, I realized, to try and insert a drip into a vein in his little ankle.

"Your son has pneumococcal meningitis" we were told. The homeopath was lurking in the background, very subdued. I ignored him. "What has he been given medicinally?" they kept asking me. "Bryonia" I stuttered. "What the hell's that?" They were very, very angry. "It's a homeopathic remedy—wild hops, I think" I said. "Wild HOPS?" they exploded.

The homeopath had disappeared.

At some moment during that morning we met the calm, quiet, serious consultant pediatrician, who told us "Your son is very, very ill. Can you find the courage not to ask me anything for a week?"

Somehow we found that courage.

It was not till a day or two later that the doctors admitted that the fact that Ben had not been on any recent antibiotic treatment would help the huge doses of antibiotics they were now pumping into him to take· maximum effect.

By then I had lost complete "faith" in homeopathy and even now, nearly forty years later, have enormous reservations about it. What fools we were to allow those days of delay which very nearly proved fatal.

On the morning he was admitted to Great Ormond Street Hospital, his heartbroken eight-year-old sister said, "Is he going to die?" And I heard myself say firmly, fiercely "NO, he ISN'T." We had the greatest difficulty in persuading her to go to school with her older sister and their friends. That night I gave her a gold painted wooden angel my dear American "mother," Louise Welch, had given me after a trip to Mexico, telling her the angel would take care of her and of Ben. She kept the angel by her bed for many years.[1]

For a week Ben lay unconscious, the doctors unable to tell us whether he would live or not.

I spent most hours of that long week with him.

Watching him emaciate before my eyes.

Watching from a distance as gowned and masked doctors and nurses again and again sought good veins into which to pump the huge doses of antibiotics.

Gently touching his hand all the time, and singing to him hour after hour his favorite nursery rhymes, which at that time were difficult to get through without crying—"Matthew, Mark, Luke and John, bless the bed that I lie on. Four angels at my bed, two at my feet, two at my head."

"Hush, little baby, don't say a word, Mama's going to buy you a mockingbird ... "

Occasionally toward the end of that long week of singing these songs, a little cracked voice, almost unrecognizable, so diminished and enfeebled it was, would demand, "Make the radio louder."

Sometimes I almost fell asleep with my head close to his on the bed ...

He came back to us slowly, slowly and miraculously without loss of hearing, sight, mobility or brain damage.

As he began to get better, his love-filled Hungarian grandmother would come, strong, calm, quiet, collected, bringing tiny tempting puddings—the ones she knew he had always enjoyed. Many years later he would tell me that was about the one thing he remembered—"Little Grannie bringing me those puddings ... "

And she would turn to me and say, "Now go! You go home and rest! I am here." And I knew I really could go with peace of mind.

One day as we were parking the car outside the hospital, I saw a little boy sitting on the balcony in the warm June sun, looking at a book. "Look at

---

1 On a recent visit to her house, where Ben's little daughter, Jenna, was staying, I was touched to see the angel placed above her bed.

that sweet little boy up there," I said to my husband. And looked again and saw it was our dear Ben in a familiar favorite green-checked shirt, his blond hair long uncut.

Among the treasures I discovered after his death I found his own account of that moment and others in the little autobiography he wrote when he was nine:

I had to go to hospital in 1972 because I had a disease called meningitis.

One thing I can remember is an African nurse giving me biscuits and cocoa at 9 p.m. One horrible thing was my EEGs, but they were quite fun really because they gave me the papers and I have still got them. And when we went for checkups we had to wait hours and on the way back we had sausage rolls. And I also remember being told that Mum said to Dad, "Look at that sweet little boy up there"; and it turned out to be me.

Even at that distance, looking up at him, I sensed his fragility and a sub-dued solemnity as if he felt cautious, precarious as he began the slow haul to regain the weight and energy of a healthy small child.

I have never forgotten the first night I watched him again in his own bed in his own room which we had redecorated in yellow ... the pain-fully thin arms flung upwards above his head, lying there flat on his back, deeply asleep, relaxed ... pain gone, fear gone, HOME again.

A few weeks later we took him and his sisters to the mountains in Switzerland, and almost the first thing he did was fall into a swimming pool. Again I found among his writings his own vivid account of what happened:

My First Experience of ... Swimming?

... My family and I were on holiday. During the day we spent most of the time at a huge swimming pool. It seemed huge to me seeing as how I was only five at the time. It was a square place filled with many exceed-ingly round women. I had imagined them to have been living off choco-late cake all their lives. (Ben and his sisters could never get over the large numbers of "pear-shaped" people in a state of bodily collapse lying by the pool.) On one side of the place, there were rectangular dressing rooms that were filled with small round men with their overpowering wives. And on the other side were round tables and umberellas [sic] sticking out of them. My Father and Mother were being joined by one of my older sisters. They were sitting at these white tables.

My other elder sister was feeling proud, as the only one of us who were [sic] daring enough as to intrude on the huge ladies making foreign noises and splashing their frilly headdresses in the swimming pool! I was playing a game with her. It consisted of her being pulled and pushed in and out of the pool—by me. As you can imagine, the procedure was bound to alter at some point. And it did. Balance failed. The concrete slabs grabbed! The water glinted with glee as I plunged to the deep end. Head first. Even now, five years later, I still recall the fixed, memorised portrait of the divided by floures-cent [sic] balls on a nylon string, pool; infected and infested by white round legs.

My sharp sister grabbed after my absence and pulled me back to surface, by my leg.

As my blue limbs crawled out of the pool, with help from my tear-shedding sister, I was greeted by my tear-shedding mother! I was draped in towels and comforted by icecream and attention.

Photos taken during that convalescent holiday show a rosy smiling little boy who had regained a normal weight and a fair degree of normal energy. Nevertheless, I think he never fully regained the energy of a very healthy child. Before this illness he had plenty. He was not wild, but full of the enjoyment of the physical activity natural to a fit child—running here, running there. Splashing around in paddling pools and charging about with his friends.

In December 1980, aged 13, Ben was diagnosed with severe, extensive ulcerative colitis.

Amid the hurly burly of family life I had nevertheless dimly registered somewhere in the back of my mind that he seemed to be going to the lavatory rather more often than usual.

One evening I found it unflushed and with a considerable amount of blood in it.

It didn't take long to establish who had last used it. And it didn't take me long either to understand this was a child's way of telling me something embarrassing and scary.

I was alarmed and took him to the doctor the very next day.

Yes, I confirmed, he had been losing weight over the past few months, but I had put it down to the rapid growth of a thirteen-year old.

Diagnosis was swift. I had no idea what ulcerative colitis really was. I was told an appointment would be made for Ben to see a gastroenter-ologist.

Meanwhile, various dietary restrictions were advised.

It was only when I told a doctor friend of the diagnosis, and she explained properly just what ulcerative colitis was all about, that I began to take on board that Ben had a singularly vile and serious illness—even potentially life-threatening.

Long before the outpatient's appointment he was eventually given, Ben was admitted to hospital—the first of many, many admissions—with severe vomiting, abdominal pain and diarrhea. These were the symptoms of the colitis with which he and we were to become all too miserably familiar for a long time before it was agreed that drastic surgery was needed.

While he was in hospital he underwent numerous unpleasant tests, X-rays, examinations. When he had recovered from the attack, and was ready to be discharged, a junior doctor came up to the ward, sat Ben and me down and without any regard for Ben's age, told him that he indeed had "extensive" ulcerative colitis. He then proceeded to run through a terrifying list of all the possibilities from the relatively mild to the most extreme which Ben might, no, would undoubtedly, experience for the rest of his life: bouts, possibly frequent, of discomfort and acute illness sufficiently severe to need hospitalization. He showed us the X-rays of Ben's colon from which I could see the abnormalities of perforations, inconsistent thickness and thinness, etc.

I was so shocked by the tactless way this was being told to a child that at first I was frozen into silence, and then afraid that if I said anything it would make it clearer to Ben how serious this illness was and frighten him. Ben, for his part, sat there in a daze, as if not really taking any of it in. In fact, I don't think he *was* taking it in.

Of course he was prescribed the appropriate medications then in use, including a very low dose of steroids.

After he was home again, I went to see our GP and told him what had happened. He was outraged and arranged for Ben to be transferred into the care of another specialist at another hospital. Ben developed a very good trusting relationship with this kind man, who for nearly two years battled to keep Ben from surgery. He did indeed have many episodes where he was so very ill he had to be rushed into hospital and was more or less constantly on steroids, the doses carefully monitored but at times very high.

> Illness grasped me.
> My stomach writhed and my belly kicked.
> Hospital was my doom.
> My parents arranged a stay in Intensive Care.
> We rushed—I a newborn foal,
> Layers to hold in body heat.
> Pain and no muscle functioning properly.
> A trolley for an x-ray.
> A needle for a drip.
> Peace in a hospital bed.
>
> —1982, 14 years

In spite of all this illness and suffering, Ben bravely lived as often as possible—with no fuss or self-pity—as normally as possible. He went to school, on camping and skiing trips. He studied, he played, he made many good friends—so good that when he died some of them, over a quarter of a century later, came to the celebration of his life.

One of those friends bore witness to this in words he wrote to us when Ben died, and which are in the memory book we have made for his little daughter: *Ben was a very special person and a dear friend . . . his laugh, his smile, his subtle sense of humor, his fortitude during his illness at school. We had a lot of fun, a lot of laughs.*

Looking back it seems unbelievable that he was in hospital about every 6 weeks until it was finally blindingly obvious to everyone that this could not continue.

He was admitted in November 1982 and underwent an *ileo-rectal-anastomosis*, in other words a skillful internal solution to remove most of the colon, but which meant some diseased tissue had to be left *in situ*. The surgeon saw us after the operation and told us that Ben's colon looked like a chewed up piece of string.

He made an astonishingly swift and good recovery and for the next ten years or so lived a full and action-packed life with all the confusions, ups and downs, and adventures normal for a young adult: girl-friends, a first true love, traveling all over Europe and even making a never-to-be-forgotten trip to Australia and Tasmania.

It was during this time that he developed his outstanding gift for photography which had begun early on during convalescent periods of his illness, and had led to the establishment of his own dark room in the old coal cellar under our house and enormously valued moments of sitting at the feet of two outstanding photographers—one being no less than our neighbor, Fay Godwin.

He completed his sixth form education and went on to study History at Bristol University ending with a 2.1 in spite of having devoted a huge amount of his time to a new found passion—theater! He was soon acting, directing, designing and putting on shows at Bristol and more than once at the Edinburgh Festival. I can see him now flinging himself about with complete joyful abandon in the singing and dancing line of *Guys and Dolls* and feeling partly anxious, but mostly delighted, to see him able to take part so fully in something so energetic. And just as he had made true friends at school, he made many more now with

whom he would stay close—and later with their wives and children—
for the rest of his life: good, good friends who would prove a bastion
of love and support to us all when he died—one coming as soon as
she could from New Zealand after his first cardiac arrest, and again in
August 2006 to be present at the burial of his heart, who, as we stood
at the grave told us how she had until recently always thought of Ben as
her "little brother" but had come to feel that he had become indeed her
"big brother" full of wisdom and experience.

———

And then, suddenly, in 1992 he had his first bout of "ITP" or *idiopathic
thrombocytopenic purpura*—a rare auto-immunological blood disorder
where the platelet count drops dangerously low for unknown reasons
and there is hemorrhaging—in Ben's case from the diseased rectal tissue. He was to have two more of these episodes over the next ten years,
always sudden, always necessitating blood transfusions—2 or 3 bags
full, followed by months of high steroid dosage, gradually tapered off
and stopped. During the first episode he seems to have had some kind
of 'near death experience' which he described to me later –"I sort of
passed out, Mum, and it was bliss . . . a sort of letting go, no struggle, not
frightening . . . " Had he been swept a little way on that "cosmic wave,"
that "cosmic impulse" which Sri Anirvan[1] describes in his piece *Life-
Death?*[2] I am inclined to believe that this brief moment, this profound
impression of another state was the foundation for his attitude from
then on toward death. "I'm not afraid of dying," he would tell his sister,

---

1   Sri Anirvan (1896–1978)—a Bengali spiritual seeker, scholar and teacher in the
    Samkhya tradition.
2   The moment of physical death or of passage to a lighter density . . . is a moment of
    transubstantiation, a function of the spirit (*Purusha*) informed by sensation (*Sakti*).
    When you are face to face with death, do not struggle. Let yourself glide. The wave
    that will carry you away is cosmic. (Sri Anirvan quoted by Lizelle Reymond in *To
    Live Within*, her account of the five years she spent with him as a student, practicing
    the discipline he taught which he called "yoga in life".)

Lucy, during the last year of his life, "but I am afraid of having to say good-bye." Thank God he was to be spared that pain.

I remember going to see him after he had been admitted to hospital, and being barely able to distinguish where his face ended and his pillow began due to his extreme and alarming pallor . . .

I remember too the cheerfulness as he lay there intravenously hooked up to the transfusion, drips in other veins, always positive, always gracious, always grateful to the doctors, the nurses and us for visiting him.

After the first episode he, of course, had to present himself regularly at the Hematology Unit to have his platelet count monitored. And after each checkup he would thoughtfully phone me to give the good news that it was once more normal. One of his first questions when he came round from the first cardiac arrest in July 2005 was, "Mum, is my platelet count all right?" and sank back relieved to sleep when I was able to confirm that the doctors' response was "Yes, it is."

In spite of this new threat—he knew that it could happen again (and it did)—Ben continued to live to the full. After a spell in various media-orientated jobs including a stint in a TV production company, followed by a well-paid job making educational CD-ROMs, his interest turned again to theater and to design in particular. Inspired by working for a while backstage for Opera North and also as one of the stage managers for a production of two poignant operas by courageous composers in Terezin for the children of Terezin[1] (from where they would be sent to Auschwitz), he decided to do a degree in stage design at the Wimbledon School of Art. Among the many treasures I found after his death are some of his immensely well researched and beauti-

---

1 The concentration camp masquerading as an ideal town for Jews to live in, 30 km from Prague and where Ben's paternal great-grandmother perished in 1944.

fully written essays on theater history, stage design, as well as his own eloquent thoughts and ideas. I had no idea just how much he had read during those years—and widely read in his usual eclectic searching way. And I was deeply touched when I came across letters from his tutors, acknowledging how hard he was working in the teeth of ever-present poor health which included a second episode of ITP. They were understanding enough to allow him extra time to complete the degree course which indeed he did.

—

The last of these ITP episodes was not long after he met the lovely woman he was to marry. He seemed to enter a golden moment of very great happiness and the imminent promise of fulfillment professionally as well as in his personal life. His health seemed improved: it was even suggested to me by a doctor that he was not surprised to hear this since surely his joy and satisfaction in all domains would "strengthen his immune system." Yes, well . . .

In 2002 he and Vicky came shyly round to tell me that they were going to get married. A couple of years before that Ben had added the PGCE[1] to his other degrees. He had decided to qualify as a teacher after a year or more of worthwhile, interesting hands-on work in schools all over the country.[2] Perhaps this was where his genuine interest in children and his natural sympathy for and empathy with them came vividly into being. But yet again he was to be stymied by his health, finding daily classroom teaching simply too physically demanding. He looked for other ways to use his skills with children which led to a stint at the Ancient Technology Centre in Dorset, where he helped to build their famous Earthhouse as well as working in many varied ways with

---

1 Postgraduate Certificate of Education, an extremely taxing one-year course.
2 Working for the late Nigel Frost who had come up with the inspired way of teaching children how to make three dimensional forms by the simple use of sticks and rubber bands to build their own designs.

groups of visiting schoolchildren. Again in time this job also proved too strenuous. He worked for a while in London at School Works,[1] where he began to deepen his concern about the effect, more often than not undesirable, of unsatisfactory school buildings and school spaces. From there he went to the taxing job as "mentor"[2] in a tough primary school, once again enjoying the direct if demanding contact with children. Gradually the strands were coming together and he realized that his "passions" were children in education and their real needs if they were going to have a beneficial time at school. He was making more and more contacts and friends within the world of "alternative" schooling. He began writing articles, and was pondering on where to go next when suddenly he was "headhunted" to become the first director of "Shape."[3]

Add to all this the many projects and adventures he undertook at snatched moments between employment to work in the forests of Oregon, the Kentish woods, learning how to build straw bale houses, cob building, wood crafts, or trekking alone up the West Coast of the USA sleeping on fabulous beaches, making friends wherever he went, visiting schools in California and—the high point of it all—spending ten days on the John Muir Trail in the Sierras, and the picture emerges of an exceptionally gifted young man searching in many places and in many forms for his right place, the place where he could bring together all his studies, all his labors, all his interests, all his experiences, all his gifts in order to serve in some worthwhile way, and at the same time attain a sense of fulfillment which would never mean resting on his laurels.

And so, during the famous heat wave of 2003, came a beautiful wedding

---

1 School Works is a design initiative to raise educational achievement in secondary schools. Ben helped to oversee the development of a socially deprived school.

2 A mentor's job is to work one-to-one with any child whose pastoral or learning difficulties are having a negative effect on their education.

3 Now Shape East, the Architecture Center in Cambridge which engages the public in issues affecting the local built environment with a particular focus on arousing children's and young people's interest and concern in these matters.

ceremony in an ancient building in York—the sun shone fiercely, the sky was cloudless and a hundred guests came to rejoice in the overflowing happiness of Ben and Vicky. No-one who was there is likely to forget Ben's poetic love-letter to his wife—twenty minutes of rhapsody. It was obviously the happiest day in their lives and probably the happiest in mine—to witness the radiance of their love, the vivifyingness of their love; to rejoice that Ben at last had found the woman he was to tell both his sister and me in phone calls less than three hours before his death was "the center of his life"; the room was filled with the absolute delight and well-wishing of their many friends (some of whom had come specially from New Zealand and Australia), let alone their families, that these two had found each other and now been joined together.

The golden moment continued: they moved to Cambridge, Ben's demanding job excited and enthused him; people began to be impressed by him and his efforts and his ideas, not least his tremendous empathy with children.

And then, the crowning of their joy: the birth on 1 September 2004 of their perfect daughter, Jenna Grace.

So much happiness, so much love, so much promise radiated from this little family, embracing, including all of us, both her family and his.

Their tiny rented house now more cramped than ever with "a pram in the hall," they were very soon in the throes of looking for a house of their own when suddenly, seemingly out of nowhere, when their baby was only five months old, in February 2005, Ben fell very ill.

He manifested the all too familiar symptoms of a major flare-up of the ulcerative colitis—nausea, vomiting, diarrhea, stomach pain. Before long he was admitted to hospital and put on a drip to counteract the inevitable dehydration. Within 48 hours he seemed recovered, was up pushing his drip-stand with him, appetite back and soon after that home again. But, within barely a day or two, all the symptoms returned even more ferociously and once more he was admitted to Addenbrooke's. This time round he could not stop vomiting, retching and hiccoughing. Day after day he was bent over a bowl becoming more and more exhausted and wretched. Worryingly, he had been told that a virus had activated itself in his gut: CMV. Cytomegalovirus[1], which was severely aggravating his condition. He was prescribed powerful drugs normally used to counteract HIV and Aids. It was some time after his death that I found out more about CMV and began to wonder whether this apparent acute flare-up of the ulcerative colitis was perhaps actually not that, but this terrible virus, or whether indeed he had been assailed by CMV on top of the colitis.

It was at the height of this episode that what I can only describe as a miracle took place—a miracle[2] called down through dire, dire need.

It starts on the train on one of the many days I visited him during that time. I try to collect myself perhaps more strongly than I ever have before . . .

There he is bent double over the bowl, retching, retching, retching . . . utterly drained, despairing, tearful but without the energy to release the sobs . . .

I sit down and rest my hand gently on his back . . .

His sister, Lucy, arrives. She sits facing him on the edge of the bed. There isn't much space and our knees are touching. She rests her hand on his forehead.

So we are all connected physically and it soon becomes apparent in some other way, connected to a merciful force, a merciful energy . . .

"Let me lean on you," he says to his sister.

She arranges herself so he can rest against her shoulder.

We are all still touching . . .

I move to be in front of him so I can put compresses on his sweating

---

1 "This illness with CMV virus almost certainly involved Ben's heart from the findings at post-mortem. If so, then Ben's thick heart muscle problem was not genetic, but acquired from viral CMV damage." —Richard S. Crampton, distinguished Professor of Cardiology, University of Virginia

2 In the words of G. I. Gurdjieff "a 'miracle' can only be a manifestation of laws unknown to men, or rarely met with . . . the manifestation in this world of the laws of another world."

forehead. Lucy has brought an essence of lavender spray from Provence. We prepare compresses soaked in this and gently bathe his forehead and the back of his neck . . . all the time murmuring, not even words really, the sort of murmuring of mothers with small sick children.

Weeping now, hiccoughing, sweating, retching, then he begins to speak—'in tongues' one could say: "I love that smell of lavender. It reminds me of Vers (the remote village in Provence where he stayed as a child aged 9 and has never been back since and where, indeed, the lavender has come from). It reminds me of Bernard (the old friend in whose house we had been staying all those years ago). How is he? I love Bernard . . . I see Joanna (his godmother who died in 1994) at her funeral . . . She's dancing, dancing up, up, upwards . . . I see a blue Buddha (he didn't know until I told him much later that in Tibetan Buddhism the blue Buddha is the Medicine Buddha) . . ."

We murmur responses—affirmative responses and continue with the compresses. All this time all three of our bodies are touching each other.

He quietens. He stops weeping. He stops retching. He stops hiccoughing.

"I am tired . . ."

We move each side of the bed and gently lower him down onto the pillows, still with a compress on his forehead. His eyes close. We put the sick bowl close to him. We stand there watching him for a while. It is quite obvious that he has fallen into a very deep sleep.

We creep away to the coffee shop downstairs and stare at each other. Dumbstruck.

We get tea and coffee.

We are incoherent with barely voiced questions . . .

Something happened. God! Something happened . . .

We wait for about an hour before returning to the ward, and find him lying fast asleep exactly as we left him.

We leave, after drawing a kind doctor's attention to his peacefulness and the fact that he has not vomited anymore . . . hasn't stirred for over an hour. The doctor reassures us he will be watched carefully.

We go home on the train. Numb. Silent. Eyes closed, tears pour down his sister's face.

At home I break down as I try to tell his father what has taken place.

Next morning Vicky phones us from his bedside to tell us he is much, much better, sitting up in bed, eating rice crispies.

Quite soon after that he was discharged . . .

Out of his deep, deep need and our whole-hearted response to it a contact must have been made with a very fine, healing energy.

———

His gastroenterologist visited him often. I was there one day when he came to see Ben with a surgeon. They told him that the first task was to get him better—which they could do, and then they must seriously consider further major surgery to ensure that he would no longer be so at the mercy of his disease . . .

At last! It seemed a line could soon be drawn under those long decades . . .

But it was not to be . . .

One evening in March 2005 Ben phoned me.

Not long discharged from hospital after three weeks of serious illness, he had recently been to see his gastroenterologist as an outpatient, and had also undergone a biopsy or biopsies . . .

I can no longer recall, or don't wish to recall, the precise details of what he told me that evening, but I remember how my heart sank as he began to speak about "differentiated cells," "dysplasia" and intimations of possible surgery, major surgery, within the next few months.

Yes, crouched over the phone, as if that would somehow get me closer to him, my heart sank and I had a hard time keeping my voice steady, calm, non-reactive.

Now, I see that was the beginning of it all. The beginning of the end.

In April I went up to Cambridge early one morning to wheel the baby round the Botanical Gardens while Ben and Vicky went back to the hospital for further discussions with various consultants and specialist nurses. A major operation was proposed and booked for 14 July. Something clever, something well-tried these past twenty years, involving complete removal of all diseased tissue and the forming of an internal "pouch," which, once the body had become accustomed to it, was apparently very effective in improving the quality of daily life.

A proviso had been added—that if at surgery this operation proved impossible he would have to have instead an ileostomy. They had come back with little illustrated booklets which they decided not to study yet. Ben, as usual, took all this in his courageous, positive stride. His specialist nurse soon put him in touch with a man who had had the pouch surgery and who spoke about it very positively, saying that it had indeed transformed his life: health enormously improved, he was now married with children and a good job. Ben was immensely cheered and encouraged by this conversation and the man's kind offer that he should call him at any time before or after the operation.

I asked Vicky what she thought would be the best help I could give when he went into hospital. She asked me to focus on the hospital "end," visit Ben frequently so she would always know he was being supported, while she would focus on taking care of little Jenna, fitting in her own visits round the baby's needs.

We moved into a better moment: from April until 14 July Ben was well. Able to take a little holiday to the Norfolk beaches. Able to have fun with us all, joining in a silly, hilarious treasure hunt for Easter eggs, enjoying an Easter Sunday lunch in bliss with his wife and their little girl. All photos of him during this time—and indeed even those up to very shortly before his death—show a happy, always smiling, handsome man.

On 10 July, four days before the surgery, we all had a party in Cambridge—in the garden, the baby ending up in her paddling pool, watched over by her doting father. Ben was in good spirits. It was an upbeat moment, even though behind it there was anxiety, thinking of the ordeal he would be going through before the "benefit" of it would be experienced.

He was admitted to Addenbrooke's on 13 July 2005. We spoke on the phone that evening. He had over those last past days expressed momentary anger that he had to go through this further "insult" as doctors call it, to his body. He was fed up, but once again his courage prevailed. He had told us that he would be taken after the operation into the High Dependency Unit, as he would need special monitoring after such a major intervention.

On 14 July we went up to Cambridge, timing our arrival at the hospital with the estimated time he had told us he would probably be coming up from theater.

When more than an hour had passed with no sign of him, I began to be suspicious that something had "gone wrong." A nurse phoned down to theater and came back with the information that he was in the Recovery Room, but they were waiting for his pain to settle . . .

We waited silently in the Day Room; we paced the corridor and at last saw him being wheeled out of the lift, semi-conscious and taken straight back to his bed on the ordinary ward. My heart lurched; my mother instinct immediately kicked in: things had obviously not gone to plan. What had happened? When he had been settled back in his bed, we went to him, one of us on each side of the bed. He opened his eyes and groped for our hands, holding onto them tightly.

When Vicky arrived we left and set off for their house, where her mother was looking after the baby.

We were just drawing up in front of the house when our mobile went off . . .

Ben's mother-in-law: Vicky just phoned: Come back to the hospital at once.

We turn round. At the lights, which are red, Paul says: "What can it be?"

I say, "Cancer," petrified to say out loud that he might have died . . .
Yes, cancer. Three tumors in the bowel, discovered when they began to operate.

He is amazing: "Well, I am alive. I have a lovely wife, a lovely child . . . great job . . . "

Surgeon tells us: It will be more difficult for you all, watching . . .

He is clearly very distressed.

Only a few days after he got home we all went up to Cambridge to celebrate the fact, and to make evident our support for them in all they had to face and get used to.

Everyone brought food of every kind. Ben was hungry, tucking into everything, enjoying eating again, as he always had. He seemed astonishingly well.

And was it really just the next evening, only ten days after the surgery that we get a phone call from Vicky as we are eating supper, saying he had been rushed by ambulance back to hospital, vomiting incessantly and in great discomfort?

"What could have caused that?" we are asking each other. "Something he had eaten? That mackerel pate? The tarasamalata?"

Ten minutes later the phone rings again. Vicky: "He has collapsed . . . I think you'd better come at once . . . "

Never have I moved so fast. Never. Bag, a few toiletries, night things . . . Taxi to King's Cross (thank God only ten minutes from our house).

I am there again now—in that train, sitting there speechless, urging the train on.

Taxi to the hospital. The guy is playing loud pop music. Paul asks him to turn it down a bit. He does—by a fraction. When I say, "We want the ICU", the driver says, "That'll be A & E then." "No," I say. "Not. It's the Main Entrance." Which is locked as by now it is 10:30 or even 11 p.m. We press a button, a voice answers, we explain. Door opens. We rush to lift, to ICU waiting room through endless doors, where we find Vicky. We have to wait a very long time before we can see him. Vicky phones her mother, babysitting Jenna Grace, asks her to ring round and get us into a hotel for the night.

At last we are allowed to see him, not before lathering our hands carefully at the spirit gel dispensers nowadays at every door and every bed throughout the hospital.

There he is, my son. Hooked up to myriad gadgets beeping, green lines jiggering on the monitor, red numbers appearing, registering temperature, blood pressure, God knows what else. Tubes in the belly, drains draining, the life support machine wheezing steadily, his mouth open, slack, full of this and that. And far, far away from us. Heavily sedated into an intentional unconsciousness and frozen cold to give entire system a rest.

Cardiac arrest.

Once he had been admitted they had done everything they could to stop him vomiting: to no avail.

Earlier that evening they had all been standing round his bed, doctors, nurses, trying to put a line down into his stomach to ease the vomiting spasms, when suddenly—he collapsed.

It had taken them 35 minutes to bring him out of the arrest, using every device known to them—CPR and electric shock (which was to leave him burned on his arm and with singe marks on his chest). I think we were told that there happened to be a cardiologist on the ward at the time, and that altogether if Ben had been anywhere else than where he was he would have died then and there.

Cause? At some point we were told that it was thought to be due to dire electrolyte (blood salts) imbalance—little or no potassium (which can happen if you are severely dehydrated).

We stand at the foot of the bed. When allowed to approach him, I kiss his cold, cold forehead and whisper *Love, love, love, light, light, light, my darling . . .*

I think sometimes we are standing, sometimes sitting.

Stunned. Tearless.

I remember at one moment sitting there side by side with Vicky. She put her hand on mine. There was no place for words or tears.

Silence. Focus. Love.

———

Go to hotel. Don't sleep.

Next morning, back again.

No change.

Ben's sisters come with their husbands.

We come and go in the waiting room. Only two can go to him at a time. We take turns. We sit silently. Sometimes we drink Coke or try to nibble at a sandwich. Other families come in who are going through their own great anxieties. They make tea, offer us tea. We share our worries a little. A devoted daughter curls up on two chairs for a kip.

Suddenly Lucy bursts into great sobs: "Is he going to die?"

"NO!" I say brazenly just as I had all those years ago when he had meningitis and hugging her close, close, close. No . . . No . . . No.

And so we keep watch over him for two days and two nights.

Then they tell us they are going "to start waking him up."

From the outset we had been given to understand that there was no way of telling whether he would wake up and if he did, whether he would have suffered brain damage . . .

It is on Lucy and Luke's watch that he opens his eyes.

They phone us at the B & B near Ben and Vicky's house—a haven of quiet, kindness, and cleanliness.

"He's awake! He's opened his eyes!"

We go to the ICU at once.

He is very drowsy.

I lean over and kiss him on his forehead, touch his head gently.

"Just go with the flow, darling."

He nods, eyes closed.

We go away, dazed, near to tears, then in tears, then near to tears. Exhausted, I think we went to sleep for awhile.

Lucy goes back in the night to sit with him.

I can't sleep till she gets back to us at 1 a.m.

She comes in smiling. She comes in laughing.

I can't believe my eyes.

"Mum, he is on a roll! He can't stop talking and cracking jokes! I have never heard him so funny! I expect it's the effect of all the different drugs and things. He says he is up there with Billy Crystal with his jokes. The nurses were all laughing. I said, 'Is this normal?' They said, 'Never mind what it is! He is awake and talking . . .'"

"I think I might live to be an old man, don't you, Luce? I might live to be 70 or even 80!" "And he kept saying, 'Where's Vicky? Where is Jenna?' He kept on asking the same things again and again as if he couldn't remember what I had said, so I kept telling him they were fine and at home and asleep and would come first thing in the morning . . . In the end the nurses told him he better try to calm down and get some sleep . . . They were smiling . . . You could tell they were so happy he had woken up . . ."

Very soon he is moved to the High Dependency Unit. He is hot and clammy. We take turns at bathing his forehead with cold water wipes. Lucy has the knack better than anyone. She just rests her hand firmly on his forehead. He likes that, doesn't want to be stroked. He is also very thirsty. I help him to drink water from a paper cup. The nurses love him—his courtesy, his humor; they tend him frequently.

Late evening his father and I visit him again. He holds my hand. The drugs that are wearing off are giving him not hallucinations exactly, but strange images. He's not sure if the blue Venetian blinds are blinds or Matisse cut-outs; his father's hands look like talons—"like Edward Scissorhands" . . . He is not exactly afraid of these strange images, but needs reassuring that these effects will wear off.

It is then that he looks me full in the eye and says, "Mum, I trust you. Am I dying?" And I say, "No," but I know that if he was I would have to say, "Yes" . . .

And later again, "Mum, am I getting better?" "Yes, darling. Yes, you are definitely getting better."

A few days after he is home again, his father and I take a short trip to the Fitzwilliam Museum, and I find myself in front of a Deposition painted on wood, early Italian Quattro Centro, by someone I have never heard of. Mary to the left on the narrow panel is helping her son down from the Cross. Anguish and love on her face.

"I know that. I am she. He is my son," I say to myself. "I have just done that." A painting of any mother, any child—all love, all caring, all tenderness, all sorrow.

I weep silently—with relief, for *my* son is not dead. IS NOT DEAD . . .

And as I write this, more memories well up: of Ben, one bright early spring day last year. Was it only last year?

He spots a color photo in a newspaper of Piero della Francesca's *Madonna del Parte*.

"Gosh, Mum! Look at that! Look at that face!"

He swiftly, but neatly, tears it out and sticks it onto the fridge with a child's magnet.

It stayed there for some long while after he died.

(Some years ago, a few days before Ben's godmother died, I was massaging her neck gently as she sat limply in an armchair by the window overlooking her lovely garden, the garden she herself had labored in with love and passion. Suddenly she said, "Oh, Jenny, help me! Help me! It is awful . . . "

And I heard coming through me, God alone knows from where, "The mothers are there. We are loved."

And she nodded.)

I like to think that when Ben saw that "mother" and placed that face somewhere where he would see it many times a day that the impression that face made on him never left him—by definition an impression being something pressed in, pressed upon—in this case the heart.

And this thought leads me to these remarkable words of an Ethiopian woman:

> How can a man know what a woman's life is? A woman's life is quite different from a man's. God has ordered it so. A man is the same from the time of his circumcision to the time of his withering. He is the same before he has sought out a woman for the first time, and

afterwards. But the day when a woman enjoys her first love cuts her in two. She becomes another woman on that day. The man is the same after his first love as he was before. The woman is from the day of her first love another. That continues all through life. The man spends a night by a woman and goes away. His life and body are always the same. The woman conceives. As a mother she is another person than the woman without child. She carries the fruit of the night for nine months in her body. Something grows. Something grows into her life that never again departs from it. She is a mother. She is and remains a mother even though her child dies, though all her children die. For at one time she carried the child under her heart. And it does not go out of her heart ever again. Not even when it is dead. All this the man does not know; he knows nothing. He does not know the difference before love or after love, before motherhood or after motherhood. He can know nothing. Only a woman can know and speak of that.[1]

A postscript

One of the best pieces of advice I ever received—shortly after Ben had seemingly recovered from the effects of CMV activating itself during a major flare-up of the ulcerative colitis in 2005—was from a friend whose daughter had died a most untimely death some years ago. I had often observed the beauty and discreet sorrow on her face in repose, as if she dwelt in another world—a world I never dreamed I would one day inhabit. We were sharing an umbrella on a miserably cold, wet March day, huddling at the graveside of an old mutual friend.

Suddenly she said, "If only . . . If only . . . I promised myself I would

---

1   Quoted by C. Kerenyi, the Hungarian scholar and mythologist in *Essays on a Science of Mythology*. He had found them in a book by the great German anthropologist, Leo Frobenius (1873-1973).

never go down that road . . . " Only she would have known what associations had provoked this remark, surprising me completely and perhaps herself too.

But her words must have lodged themselves firmly somewhere near the back of my mind. Little would I know that day how soon it would be—not much more than a year from then—that they would re-appear, their letters dancing dizzyingly, almost visibly. "If only. I promised myself I would never go down that road." Words which would be used again, but this time directly to me by the consultant gastroenterologist who had looked after Ben from age 13 till he moved to Cambridge in 2003, and who would be kind enough to invite us, if we so wished, to come and talk through the post mortem with him a few months after the death. "Whatever you do, don't go down the road of 'if only' . . . " Well meant, wise, oh so true, oh so almost impossible to obey.

My "if only": they had given him an ileostomy at 16 . . .

But I silence this swiftly, reflecting that I don't know what I am talking about. At 16 they left his young body without that "insult" in the medical meaning of the word. They left him outwardly intact, free of possible psychological problems; embarrassments; inhibitions . . . Hoping, I like to imagine, that as the years passed more advanced surgical skills would develop, which indeed they did, and from which it had been fully intended he would benefit on 14 July 2005.

Chapter 5

Last weeks

Every time I return to these last weeks it is like stepping onto a roller-coaster. I never cease to be completely amazed and overwhelmed by the frequency of his "ups" and "downs," how he was flung down again and again into depths of suffering and misery, only to spring up again to heights of joy, gratitude, and faith—he would get through it and emerge ready to engage once more fully in his rich life . . . And we? We his family and the friends who loved him so? We, too, were flung down and uplifted again and again. Thanks to him and his remarkable attitude, we were gulled, fooled, never imagining for a moment that death could possibly be so very near. Generous, brave, sweet, dear Ben.

March 2006

Early in March after 18 weekly sessions, his chemo was suspended for a couple of weeks. His immune system 'is knackered.'

The little family were supposed to go to Italy for a week with friends. It was quite obvious that Ben was not well enough to go, so he came to stay with us for some of that time. He rested. He worked on his computer. I made him all his favorite soups and chicken with squash dishes, and a few days after he got home, he called to say he had gained weight and the first resumed chemo "wasn't too bad."

The following week he had a CAT scan which showed "nothing carcinogenic," but two small "fungal lesions" on his lungs so they wanted to repeat the scan in a fortnight. (He had been troubled for a long time by an irritating cough, specially at night.)

The second chemo made him feel "a bit yucky."

April 2006

We went off to visit friends in Denmark, anxiety levels slightly lowered and even mildly happy, touched by the welcome and able to enjoy a delightful celebration of Paul's birthday . . .

But on our return Ben calls us to say that the current chemo has been stopped; there is to be a change: 6 treatments fortnightly to which a second chemo drug will be added. He has been told this combined treatment is the very best now available and "they" want him to have the maximum benefit. And he is to have urgently not, after all, a repeat CAT scan, but a PET scan at the Institute of Nuclear Medicine at University College Hospital, London.

I offer to accompany him and he said he would appreciate that.

He arrives from Cambridge by train, in the nick of time for his appointment and slightly flustered; we have only a very short time together. I try hard to be very quietly collected . . . he is called away into the radioactive department. There is even time to attend Mass in the hospital chapel after which I sit on until a nurse comes to tell me that Ben has left by another exit—patients are, of course, not allowed to return to the general waiting area once they have entered the radioactive area . . . and he was worried—I shouldn't wait for him as he wanted to dash back to King's Cross as quickly as possible.

He will not know the results of the PET scan for about 10 days.

During that time his father and I began to feel increasingly anxious about the possible results of the scan.

Then, suddenly, during lunch with visitors, he rings . . . NEGATIVE! There is no "glucose uptake," which apparently means no sign of malignant cells.

We are just so, so happy, so, so relieved . . . he is "in the clear"; he has gained weight; is quite well. This is what "they" were wanting, before the new onslaught.

A mixture of tears and laughter shared with our friends. And Ben is given a two week "reprieve" before starting the new chemo treatment. He comes during that time for a happy weekend visit with his little family, joined by his sister Lucy and her family in a love-filled atmosphere of huge relief, much laughter and rejoicing, celebration even.

Celebration—celebration always rated high in Ben's view of life. After he died, a Scottish family friend wrote:

> *Ben was such a truly glad person to know. His spirit soared way above the challenges he had to confront. It was he many years ago said: 'Celebrate! Never miss an opportunity to celebrate... little things... big things. Celebration is the most important thing we can do.' I do not know why were talking of whatever it was, but I heard and took his message to heart...*

May 2006

Ben went into hospital in Cambridge so "they" could set him up with a pump which would send the new chemo drugs steadily circulating for 2–3 days; when it was empty it would have to be flushed through and removed (which always brought him a huge sigh of relief) and he would have to go back and forth as an outpatient every week. They sited it just below his left collar-bone, considering this to be the safest place to protect it from being knocked about perhaps even by his 20 month-old daughter. He should have been able to go home the same day but by the time "they" had got the pump sited the Pharmacy was closed and they could not get the drugs till the morning. He phoned us, more annoyed than miserable. But we suffered for him that there had to be any setback to just getting on with it, which "they" did next day. Within forty-eight hours, Ben was "not feeling so good," and had two or three very bad days and nights. His mother-in-law came followed a few days later by his sister and her husband. The side effects did wear off during the week "off," but then he developed a throat infection which however did not stop "them" proceeding with the second treatment. I went up the day the pump came out to cook and keep him company. He even came with me to the station, diverting the cab en route to pick up a birthday present for his lovely wife. He was surprisingly all right and over the next days well enough to go out. Then he began to go down in energy and morale; but again within days his spirits lifted as they almost always did.

Looking back in memory and going through my diaries what is so striking is that in front of this seemingly never-ending rollercoaster, life went on—fully, normally for us all. We had overseas visitors to stay; Ben's father went about his architectural business, traveling overseas when necessary; and Ben himself had a meeting with his employers to discuss his return to work in September. It should be said that anticipation of that meeting did cause him great anxiety: what would be the terms? But there never seemed any doubt to any of us but that he *would* be well enough to return to work by then. Once again, he gathered himself to face the meeting and the questions. And on his return he rang me and told me how much he had been helped before he went by reading again in what could be called his "bible," the words of William Segal in his book *A Voice At The Border of Silence* in the section called *In the Marketplace* where he talks to a young friend about how not to "lose it" while going about one's daily business; how not to be overwhelmed by the enormous energy of life, outer life and its hurly burly.

> *It's a question of being open to those energies, at the same time not to be taken by them too much . . . The whole secret of life . . . is to give one's total attention to what one is doing now. . . . It all comes down to a question of being attentive, of giving one's attention to this moment, of being in touch with the body, knowing that the feet are touching the floor, and of being aware of the onset of emotion. Always being attentively watching. This watching tends to bring energy patterns together . . . Generally we come back over and over again to the necessity of being here as totally as possible, no matter what you are doing. But we do need also engagement of the outer world. We need engagement of ourselves with others, and with confrontations. Life is a question of challenge and response . . .*

And elsewhere in the conversation, when his young friend observes how much stress there is "in the marketplace," Ben was particularly struck by William Segal's response:

> Yes indeed. *The whole world seems to be under stress . . . More war, more antagonisms, more hate . . . One is compelled to defend oneself. I mean not to waste one's energy in antagonistic attitudes, but to be able to say "no" when "no" has to be said. And to say "yes," and not to be imposed upon, at the same time not to impose upon others. It was well put here:* "I know how to take my anger out of my pocket." *When I want to be angry I can. I can act angry and defend myself, but, interiorly I'm not angry. Interiorly, I am free.*

Sustained by these words, Ben told me he had tried to follow the counsel of keeping an awareness of the body, of the simple reminder of his feet on the floor and he knew it had "done" something, helped the atmosphere to shift from remote and formal, to something much more human and sympathetic.

Just as well, as the terms were not promising and he was downcast, discouraged, depressed.

Yet, once again, his remarkably robust spirit rose up and it was not long before he was looking at other possible ways to earn a living, or to supplement a living: imaginative ways, interesting ways, original ways, all creative, many to do with education.

Nowhere, nowhere was there any sign of anxiety; we all assumed he was going to be all right. The treatment was nearly over. I know that some of us realized that he would never regain complete full fine health, but then he had not had that for many, many years. I know that some of us even realized, somewhere deep down, barely admitted, that he might well not live to "a ripe old age," but I think it is true to say that it had not crossed our minds that he might die *now*, or *soon*, not even in "the foreseeable future."

How did he manage it? To activate in himself this incredibly positive, brave attitude. To say to me so often in full faith: "Mum, it's just a *thing*. It isn't everything"?

June 2006

After the third treatment (halfway there!), once the pump was out, he came to stay with us while Vicky took a little break with friends in Holland.

What a joyful time! How happy he was! How happy we all were! And the weather was glorious.

Saturday 3 June 2006

It was during this visit that an American professor friend and his wife came for coffee and croissants on a sunny Saturday morning.

On top form and opening immediately to our visitors in his usual wholehearted way, Ben was soon telling them of his time in Plum Village, the French retreat of the Vietnamese Buddhist master, Thich Nhat Hanh. In his turn our friend told Ben of encounters with some of the Buddhist teachers now living in California. Something was passing between them as they talked and we others listened—empathy in the warm kind eyes of the professor, excitement, enthusiasm radiating from Ben.

"What did you do with Thich Nhat Hanh?"

"Well, sometimes we walked with him slowly and in silence, and sometimes he played the flute to us beneath the full moon . . ."

And these words seem to be the quintessence of the long conversation which ensued on that bright morning barely two months before he died.

"And sometimes he played the flute to us beneath the full moon."
Of course, we all knew that the days there were filled with the simple tasks necessary and grounding when many people come together to meditate, to "sit" with such a spiritual master—cooking, cleaning, dishwashing in simple, basic conditions . . . But the quintessence was in those words, "Sometimes he played the flute to us beneath the

full moon..."

Almost certainly Ben had heard teachings, and certainly had sat daily in meditative silence and stillness, but what had stayed with him deeply was this lovely impression of a man of great being, humility and rigor. (I had witnessed for myself the quality of his sitting posture, a stillness born out of years of practice, sustained by the most perfectly straight, perfectly relaxed back I have ever seen) making music by the light of the moon.

Present moment, wonderful moment is Thich Nhat Hanh's most cherished teaching and one which Ben had long taken into his heart and his way of facing his life.

How can *my* "present moments" now he is dead possibly be "wonderful moments"?

Not possible. Or is it? Now, a year later, I begin to know that it is possible because each time I do come to myself—into the reality of the present moment—it is wonderful to be offered again and again a completely different perspective on life: a brief moment, a flash of "no-thing-ness," of is-ness—just that moment, no more, no less . . . just *playing the flute beneath the full moon*—complete, perfect moment, no words, no words. The is-ness is what had stayed in Ben from the flute playing.

And also a year later I had a sudden insight into a new understanding of the meaning of the word "Now." That it has nothing whatsoever to do with a time concept and, likewise, nor has "present moment, wonderful moment." (Bizarre that we use in this context a "time" word to describe experiences outside time . . .) They are outside time and yet can be experienced simultaneously with the "now" in time, the "present moment" in time. I saw that I have always seen those moments while sitting when light comes down, and a communication established with something much higher, much finer, as separate from my "ordinary," my outer life, and they are not—they are going on at the same time, but outside time. For some reason I found this hugely comforting, encouraging and hopeful of a different way of living with this terrible grief.

And, of course, these moments are eternally love-filled.

Early summer 2007

I go with Paul to the beautiful country churchyard where Ben is buried close to his greatly loved paternal grandparents. We have come to take photos of their headstone and measurements too so that we can give the master carver of Ben's headstone some idea of the height and width we envisage.

We pause at Ben's grave and I weep. It is raining a little. I find my way to the one bench at the top of the churchyard and watch Ben's father taking precise measurements of his parents' headstone; not for the first time, I appreciate the slender sensitive hands, the care, the calmness. My gaze moves, dazed, unbelieving, between the two graves—our beloved son's and that of my loving, forgiving parents-in-law, and sitting there in disbelief once more that Ben is really dead, my heart suddenly fills with an immense tenderness, gratitude. *Present moment, wonderful moment*—the words are suddenly there in mind and heart. And I can say "Yes" to them . . .

But that day when he told our visitors about the flute was to be one of the last lovely, happy ones. The rollercoaster was about to go into overdrive.

I can single out two more joyful days.

Sunday 3 June

Ben, his father, and I met his sister, Katy, and her husband at a crowded, pleasantly noisy Greek restaurant in Primrose Hill for lunch. The sun shone and it was warm. Ben was still in very good form and as always first and foremost interested in everyone else, how they were, what they had been doing. He enjoyed the meal. I was so intensely aware, sitting next to him, of his joie de vivre, the love that always seemed to radiate from him during those few golden years of marriage and fatherhood—a very happy, fulfilled man. We left the young ones who went walking on Primrose Hill. Some hours later Ben came back, having walked all the way *and* bought and relished an ice cream. "But now I'm knackered," he said and went off for a good, long sleep.

Could this really have been barely four weeks before he died?

Once again, looking through my diary I constate how blissful was our ignorance: every page crammed with the events and appointments of a busy life, and if I turn to his e-mails sent between March and mid-June, they are filled with joy, love, gratitude for the smallest things.

I have them all still on my computer, all of them include lovely photos of little Jenna, her mother, himself on happy outings:

20 March 2006:

Dear Ma & Pa, very glad to say I am feeling relatively okay and have eaten and drunk well tonight: thanks for the fantastic juicer you got us!!! Thank you again for the vitamins and the Supersalve: lifesavers—both!! Thought you might enjoy these pictures of my beautiful girls in Italy . . . I'll speak to you again soon. Lots of love from all of us. Bxxxx

22 March 2006:

Subject: Jenna and Vicky in Italy:

Just got up from a very long sleep and am looking forward to some juicing! Feel well rested and not too bad—a bit chesty.

Sorry you're not feeling too well. Here are some more pictures of Jenna Grace to cheer you up! Much love, B & Vxxxx

1 April 2006:

Subject: Jenna and "Dad" at Wimpole today:

Dearest Ma, Pa & Luce, We just got back from a lovely day at Wimpole Hall looking at lambs, tractors and "daffs" (as Jenna now says) . . . beautiful Spring weather nice enough for us all to have a lovely picnic. Jenna giggling for England, chatting and singing to herself.

I'm feeling good—a bit sleepy after a night out at the movies last night! (First time, for me, in ages I've been to a cinema . . .)

Give us a ring later today. It'd be nice to catch up. Lots of love, Ben, Vicky and Jenna Grace xxx

5 April 2006:

Subject: Thanks for:

Dear Ma. I tried to ring, but it was engaged . . .

Thank you so much for all the yummy food—our chicken supper was DELICIOUS! And doubly appreciated by us both as poor Vix returned from work with a cracking migraine from her very hot (dehydrating) office! (She's fine again now—and has gone to Sainsbury's) It was lovely of you to come with supplies and to cook yesterday—I really appreciate (d) it. Come again soon! It's really good to have lots of yummy leftovers and your soup. We all three had a good night last night . . . and such a lovely morning with Jenna: she is so affectionate and funny. It is quite incredible how much inspiration she gives us (and me, in this time of need). So I feel pretty good this morning, but am going back to bed for a snooze . . .) (I spoke to Luce who will come on Friday and maybe also do some yummy cooking). Speak very soon . . . Lots & lots of love, B & V xxx

11 April 2006:
Subject: Noodle drop:
dear Ma good to talk to you last night . . . what a business this strange narrative is! Thank you so much for the lovely noodle drop which I picked up this morning: much appreciated!

Speak to you soon again. Much love, Ben.
P.S. The Malevich[1] card is GORGEOUS TOO! XXX

11 April 2006:
From: "Jenny Koralek"
To: "Ben Koralek"
Subject: Re: Noodle drop:
Glad the noodles dropped in but sorry you had to go and fetch.
Yes . . . a strange narrative . . . I am with you all the way . . . Henri used to say to me at times when you were ill long ago "I am with you, and YOU are with him." No more . . . it says it all . . . and I say it to you now . . . NOW is where we try to be again and again and again. NOW and nowhere else . . . I go away from now, but I can come back . . . I AM WITH YOUxxxxxxxxxx

---

1 I had sent him one of Malevich's least abstract paintings—of children at play.

18 April 2006:
Subject: Re: Noodle Drop:
Dear Mum, I am SO moved by your thoughts and feelings expressed here. I honestly am lost for words.

But the view of NOW which you and Henri T express so beautifully—the present moment—is something that I hold to be true and very important and helps me a lot. I am keeping a copy of Thich Nhat Hanh's "Present Moment—Wonderful Moment" close by and re-reading the beautiful ghatas which are like drinking the purest mountain water in the middle of a chemical-industrial wasteland . . .

Jenna too—a little Buddha in her own right—helps me to stay in the here & now a bit more than usual. She is such an inspiration!

23 April 2006:
Subject: Lovely Sunday:
Dear Ma & Pa, thank you for a very jolly day and DELICIOUS lunch (and lovely blue/green jumper for Jenna—she looks SO cute in it). She sat in the car all the way home playing with "baby" and its pink outfit, scoffing Marmite sandwiches ("sammitch" as she says) and reciting her role [sic] call of her special people: you all! She was still burbling away when we put her to bed . . . what a sweety; and a good sign that she'd had a really good day.

I really do appreciate having your lovely soups to see me through the next few days—they'll be just the ticket I know.

And I just want you both to know that I/we really feel your loving support through everything—and I know I will feel it tomorrow at the hospital. So thank you for that too. It makes all the difference.

Lots of love, as always, B, V & Jxxxx.

08 May 2006:
Subject: Hello and lots of love and gratitude:
Hello Mum & Luce (& Luke)—lots of love to you both.

The phone's very busy today with Vicky's work stuff so I thought I'd just e-mail you both to let you know I am feeling good today: no nausea and much less tiredness (I had a long sleep this morning 'til lunchtime). Eating well, shaved and dressed! And expect to be okay to look after Jenna tomor-row PM; but if you feel up to it Mum, it would be lovely to see you, but don't feel you have to come if it's all too much.[1]

Thank you both so much for putting your minds to helping Vicky, Jenna and I in the weeks to come. [his chemo treatment about to be changed]. It

---

1   How glad I am that I went! Such a sweet May day:

    We fetch Jenna from the child carer. Proudly he carries her high in his arms. Gently installs her in the car seat, produces a drink and a little packet of California Sun Raisins she calls "rainers." "Shall we show Gummy our country way home?" "Es...," munch, munch. And we go the back way down cow-parsleyed narrow wind-ing roads, their minute undulations described by Ben as "the nearest thing we have to hills round here." *Present moment, wonderful moment* in those words of Thich Nhat Hanh which meant so much to Ben. As I write I relive the joy in him, the fulfillment, the sheer pleasure of that moment for father, daughter, mother/grand-mother just tooling along on an ordinary day, chemo pump out and hey! Just weeks away from taking that out for the very last time. Later in the warm afternoon we go walking along their road, ambling, Jenna running into other people's gardens to pick up gravel, point at butterflies and smell flowers: all "bu'bells" to her. Eventu-ally she begins to tire and Ben lifts her up on his shoulders: one happy little girl. A young woman cycles past and pauses when she sees us; calls out: "Ben! How *are* you? He greets her warmly by her name: "I didn't know you lived round here!" She cycles on and he tells me she is one of the lovely nurses who took such good care of him after his cardiac arrest last July. We wander home and out into the garden with toys and snacks on a rug. "BIG hug, Daddy!" Jenna suddenly demands. "Big hug! *Sofa*!" She is remembering the many times she and her father cuddle on the sofa in their sitting-room and is clearly telling him they must now go indoors and do that. "No," says Ben, "We can't do that—the sofa lives indoors..." "Sofa *here*," she orders. "Can't bring sofa out here," says her Daddy, "but we can still have a BIG HUG," and Jenna lunges herself into his arms and his inviting cross-legged lap. Oh, sweet May day.

    Months after his death I found Ben's copy of Gaston Bachelard's *The Poetics of Space*, a beautiful book about, among other things, the metaphysical, the almost mystical meaning of different forms of space, including the body and the house, the home. There are many underlinings, but this is the one which touches me most and seems to sum up the sense of his well-being on that May day: "Being reigns in a sort of earthly paradise of matter, dissolved in the comforts of an adequate matter. It is as though in this material paradise, the human being were bathed in nourishment, as though he were gratified with all the essential benefits."

clearly will be a different chapter in the story. I am really feeling your support right now and that counts for A LOT! (to all of us) . . .

29 May 2006:
Subject: Fun with Jenna:
Dear All, just a little Jenna update and to let you know that we have all had a lovely weekend of fun with Cambridge friends, Jenna discovering beetles, ladybirds, spiders, "fuff-flies" (butterflies) at very close range, playing with other little ones, fun in our garden (we now have a nice little round table and four chairs for sunny breakfast mornings . . . and I built a little mini greenhouse for some of our little veggies we are planting now: carrots, courgettes, squash, beetroot) . . . and as you can see from the photo we had a fab day at Wimpole today with Jenna . . . playing on mini tractors, petting the tiny ("tiner") pygmy goats and adventuring down a little slide all on her own . . .

13 June 2006:
Subject: Jenna in London & naked painting!! (and 'Hommage to Moholy Nagy (photo)
Dear Mum, Dad, Luce & Luke, some of our latest pictures of Jenna in London (Sunday morning in the playground) having a lovely time! And painting in the garden back at home. And here's the photo of the sunlight on the wine glasses I mentioned (inspired by our visit to the Moholy-Nagy/Albers show, Dad).

Not feeling too bad . . . tired, but have eaten well tonight—SO looking forward to having the pump disconnected tomorrow. And to seeing you all at the w/end . . . Lots of love all round xxxx Ben"

14 June 2006 (his 39th birthday)
To: Lucy . . . Cc to Jenny . . .
Subject: "Hommage to Moholy-Nagy" + butternut squash sprouts!!
. . . lovely to catch up with you today. Thank you again for the lovely card (I had a good crop of cards, this year, a lovely chat with Gord . . . [his best man, and who would be one of the four to carry the coffin two months later], a very jolly chat with cousin Joe who is still keen for us cousins to have a big

get-together sometime . . . all very heartening. Here are some photos for you showing our creativity and life-force bursting out all over: Jenna's first cooking (birthday cake for daddy) . . . and . . . our squash sprouts!! Aren't they cute!!' Much love, Ben xx

My diary for 14 and 15 June records "Ben not very good" (on top of which Jenna was developing chicken pox). But once again he "bounced" back—by Saturday 17 June: "Ben much better" and the little family arrive for a long weekend visit to celebrate his birthday.

He does not look wonderful. Grey complexion, the poor arm veins and palms deeply stained from the chemo drugs, eyebrows and lashes almost vanished . . . but his cheerfulness overrides everything else.

A heat wave was raging and would continue to do so well into July. We set up the paddling pool for little Jenna now visibly "poxy" but not yet miserable with it.

And there in our garden on 18 June we celebrated Ben's birthday with a *"déjeuner sur l'herbe"* joined by Lucy's family. Sadly, Paul was away, but we were merry, relaxed, lovingly engaged . . .

That evening Ben encouraged Vicky to go out to a party—he and I would babysit. He ironed her dress for her, admired her beauty, kissed her and sent her on her way.

No sooner had we settled down for a peaceful evening than Ben began to complain of a very sore mouth . . . we knew that one of the side effects of the chemo drugs he was on was mouth ulcers. And then . . .

Jenna wakes up crying her heart out—the chicken pox has really taken hold. Ben goes bounding upstairs to her.

I follow.

He is sitting on a chair, cradling her, hot, sweaty, itchy, murmuring soothingly, so sorry for her.

"Oh, Mum! Isn't she lovely!"

He asks me to fetch a spoon so he can give her some Calpol.

I help him get a teaspoon down, but that is all I am allowed to do . . .

He shelters his child beneath the "protecting veil" his friend, Robin, will speak of one day. He radiates his unconditional love for her.

Never mind that his mouth is beginning to give him severe pain. His love and care completely supersede his own suffering.

I leave father and daughter with a great ache in my heart.

———

By the time they all got home the next day, Jenna was really very ill and so was Ben. The mouth ulcers had developed rapidly and savagely and he was in terrible pain, could barely speak or eat . . . For the first time during this long cruel haul he was irritable. Vicky's mother went to help them. Later she told me she had never seen Ben so despairing . . .

Yet on four days later he was emailing us as brightly and bravely as ever:

Thursday 22 June 2006:
Subject: Thursday.
Dear Ma, Pa, Luce, just to say that I'm feeling brighter today. My mouth's still sore, but I have more energy. I've been out in the garden looking after our tomatoes and squash sprouts with Angela and Jenna in the sunshine which is lovely. I've also been deeply inspired—last night—by reading my books on Albers and (I hope you don't mind Dad but I borrowed your) Paul Klee catalogue. (I also had a chat with our neighbor about taking down our naff pine trees, to clear way for a shed, and he was absolutely fine about it, so . . . a small but important step closer to the art studio/office!)

I've also had some very lively and humorous, drug-fueled dreams: one bit from last night included me writing a really hilarious (of course) episode of "Friends"—I even woke myself up laughing at the punchline to my episode, albeit at 5 a.m.!

Jenna's spots are starting to clear too and she is more like her usual self . . . Much love, and speak (mumble) soon. Ben xxxx

———

And so, unknowingly, we were entering the last two weeks of his life.

He went back to the hospital where they prescribed very strong pain relief.

For a few days he was a little better—able to speak on phone more or less normally.

And still we all continued our lives obliviously. The end of the treatment was so very, very near now. Soon it would all be over and we would all be able to focus on helping Ben regain strength. A good holiday, we all agreed, would be top priority. Good food, tender loving care and . . .

He seemed quite a bit better. Even went out to lunch at Grantchester with a good friend where they discussed Ben's professional future— what direction that might take. He phoned me almost bubbling again with new ideas, encouraged by the discussion he had had over that meal.

The heat wave was cranking up by now and I was desperately trying to recover from a bladder infection, on antibiotics, fretting that I was not well enough to go up to Cambridge. But on Sunday 2 July his sister Lucy did go with a good friend and kept him company while Vicky went off to take part in a run for a charity devoted to cancer research.

That evening Lucy phoned me in tears . . .

"Mum, I'm really worried. He looks so ill . . . He is so tired . . . "

I decide to go up the following day, but early on that Monday 3 July Vicky phones. Ben has been admitted to Addenbrooke's severely dehydrated . . . diarrhea, vomiting, stomach cramps and jaundiced . . . and as so often before, the electrolytes seriously out of balance . . . so, of course, on a drip to remedy that as well as antibiotics . . .

The following morning his father and I go to see him . . .

Incredible turnaround!

There he is, sitting on the bed, dressed in grey t-shirt and shorts, reading Maya Angelou's *I Know Why the Caged Bird Sings*.

"Mum, Dad, you needn't have come!" Gently reproachful.

"I'm much better! I should think I'll be discharged by tomorrow . . . "

Lulled by the magic of modern medicine's capacity to correct certain disorders swiftly and effectively, we too thought it likely . . .

But he looked grey and yellowish; hot and clammy.

I had brought some strips of old sheet and went several times to the washbasin in the corner of the ward to run under the cold tap, squeeze out and give him to mop forehead and neck.

He is cheerful, wanting to talk, asking his father about work . . .

I show him the photos of his last visit to us. We laugh over Jenna hiding her eyes, thinking this meant none of us could see her; a chicken-poxy backview of Jenna stepping into the paddling pool, holding my hands, her face turned up to mine, laughing; Jenna in a huge pair of sunglasses. We smile over a sweet one of him hugging her.

I don't remember anything extraordinary about our words—affectionate, slightly upbeat, assuming soon he would be rehydrated and home again.

The one thing he *did* say to me when we were alone—when his Dad had gone downstairs to find some sandwiches for us: "Mum, I am going to ask my oncologist to let me off the last chemo . . . "

Yes, there was only one more to go . . .

I felt relief and a certain confidence that she probably *would* let him off the last pump filling, pump washing-through palaver, the days of extreme discomfort—surely one *less* out of the 39 or so he had had could not possibly make much difference? He needed to stop that now and turn toward recuperation, recovery, rebuilding his energy.

He had recently sent a long detailed e-mail to a doctor friend who had offered to put him in touch with a specialist pharmacist who could prescribe tailor-made vitamin and mineral supplementation, saying in effect, *Any day now I will be finished with the chemo and I would really welcome guidance on how to help my body recover.*

———

We stayed less than two hours, not to tire him. He was ready for a sleep when we left.

I kissed him.

He kissed me.

And as I left the ward, thank God I turned round and waved to him. He waved back.

The last time . . .

Next day: *Don't come today. Am having a CAT scan. They want to look at those fungal lesions they spotted on my lungs when I had that PET scan in April* . . .

———

I discussed visiting plans with Vicky. We would go again soon if he didn't get home. And for when he *did* get sent home she and I began to sketch out by e-mail who would come and when, to help her by being with him when she was at work. Lucy would help with that too over the weekends when *she* wasn't at work.

I still have that complex, well worked-out program on my computer.

———

Thursday 6 July evening.

I was supposed to go out to a meeting with his father, but some deep instinct, a deep unease, made me decide to stay at home. We agreed that we should not both be out in case he called.

And he *did* call: I don't remember where I was in the house, but he left a message, voice resigned, disappointed, rather low: "Bit of a bummer, Mum. They want me to have a broncoscopy and to stay in for another two weeks to treat the lesions with intravenous antibiotics. Can you phone me back? Am running out of credit on my phone thingy."

I phone back some time between 8 p.m. and 8:30.

He sounds very low and disheartened, but, overriding his own distress at not being able to go home, and the prospect of more invasion of his body, more time in hospital, is his concern for his wife and child . . .

"Mum, will you help them? I've talked to Lucy about working out some system between you to support them through this. Vicky is very understandably fed up.

Take care of her, Mum. She is the center of my life."

From the depths of my heart I reassure him, promise him that we will do everything we can to help her.

And soon we say good-bye: "Speak to you tomorrow, Mum . . . "

———

A few minutes past midnight, into 7 July, that little black phone by our bed rings: He has had another cardiac arrest.

Not long after Ben's recovery from the first cardiac arrest, I told our doctor what had happened. Although he tried to hide his reaction when I told him it had taken 35 minutes to bring him out of it, I sensed shock and gravity.

He told me sometimes cardiac arrest could occur while trying to put a line down into the stomach . . .

But then he said, "I don't mean that you should be looking out your black armband, but . . . "

I got such a shock I almost succeeded in not hearing the words.

But went out in a terrible daze, out into the street. NO, NO, NO, I will not let those words linger in me ANYWHERE, and succeeded so well I didn't tell Ben's father what the doctor had said until long, long after Ben had died, because I had completely forgotten about it.

Chapter 6

Celebration

Three months after Ben died, his wife, Vicky, organized with immense skill and all-encompassing thought and attention to detail, a superb celebration of his life. It took place on a mild and bright October day in Cambridge at the Michaelhouse Café, a perfect venue in what was once a church.

Vicky had prepared a lovely invitation with photographs of Ben's earlier years, but above all as a husband and father as well as ones showing him at work with children in schools.

The text she had written to accompany it shone out with her pride in him and of her love for him:

> Welcome to a celebration of Ben's life. Please join us . . . in remembering Ben's warmth, humor and incredible passion for life. Everything he did, he approached with one hundred percent enthusiasm from creating architectural models with children, to designing theater stage sets, from taking photographs of the wild Oregon coastline, to capturing the places he loved on canvas.
>
> Ben was a unique person. A one-off. He was always full of dreams and projects. But most of all he was a truly wonderful human being. And the world was a better place for his presence in it.

Over 200 people came—of all ages from babies to 90 year olds and from all moments of his life, professional and personal: his family and Vicky's, many lifelong friends of his parents and his sisters, who had all known and loved Ben; godchildren and school friends; former employers and Buddhists for whom he had done fundraising for projects in Mongolia, one of whom, the very gifted Michael Ormiston[1] performed Mongolian music and Khoomii (overtone) singing.

An archway of "sticks and bands" had been built to which we all added our own sticks.

There was an exhibition of many of his fine photographs; of his paintings and writings and his exquisite little sculptured figures.

We had prepared a book which we left open in the little side chapel, containing the many tributes to him which we had received when he died, and with plenty of empty pages for more to be added if anyone wished (which they did), with the purpose of collecting them all for Jenna Grace to read one day.

Everyone who read the book was struck, as we had been, by the very noticeable use of the same words, again and again, to describe impressions and feelings about Ben; so much so, it was impossible not to believe in the widely shared perception of him, which we all found very heartening and consoling, showing as it did that we were far from alone in seeing him and loving him the way we did and do . . .

. . . I think the word is a kind of radiance—a light that always was—and is—Ben . . . bright, joyful and with a completely infectious magnetism of enthusiasm and fun and twinkle and playfulness, so that everyone was pulled into the wake of his magic . . . that amazing smile. I feel to have been truly blessed that he touched my life.

I can always see his smile very clearly . . .

His patient fortitude and that wide, engaging smile . . .

A very special person.

Re-reading his letters, I am struck by his brilliance, intelligence, wit, sensitivity,

---

1   Britain's foremost Mongolian Khoomii singer.

erudition, maturity at only eighteen years . . . I wish my children might find such companions in their life to come. You equipped him so well with strength, security, spirituality and humor for his special life. And he shared it with others. Thank you.

He carried the burden of illness with such lightness and grace, and his very being exuded a golden, life-enhancing quality that seemed to banish the shadow that hung over him . . .

. . . a wonderful, funny friend.

. . . fair clean clear beautiful sweet light. Was thinking about his smile this morning.

With Ben what you see is what you get.

. . . one of the very kindest, most sweet-natured and sensitive people I have ever known. He really did stand out as someone of rare decency and gentleness. You have told us of the courage he has shown throughout his illness, without a trace of self-pity; quite the contrary—for the sake of others. How many other lives there must be which are better for having known him.

His Ben-ness will live on in Jenna . . .

My memories of Ben are of his gentleness and friendliness, both qualities I admire enormously in people. I distinctly remember his engaging smile.

. . . such a lovely man—kind, clever, artistic and interested in so much.

. . . he has borne everything with great grace and courage. I have been very affected by his good example.

Ben was brilliant with my students—he was inspirational.

. . . a lovely person—an all-round delightful, humorous and happy human being, always ready with a smile and friendly greeting. I hope you can feel proud, amidst all the sorrow, to have brought into the world someone who engendered and obviously gave such love and happiness to those around him.

. . . such an alive, cheery, fantastic person . . .

Ben absolutely LIVED, didn't he? He was so open to new experiences, so positive, so loving and so funny. I know that I have always been affected and inspired by his idealism and love of beautiful things . . . I will never forget his passionate attitude to things that interested him, and I absolutely know how much that attitude has inspired me my whole life. He was the most wonderful uncle.

Such a "golden" person, and so full of light and humor and, above all, life.

It was a happy time when I was with you when he was a young boy with a lovely smile . . . and later, when I saw him, he was always so sweet and kind.

The way I remember him—somehow delicate, but full of shine and kindness and dreams and projects.

Ben was a man I feel so blessed to have met and to have shared some of his life . . . He was so kind, so loving, so devoted—full of wonderful ideas and inspiring to observe when he was sharing them and the things he was passionate about. The world is a little darker without him . . .

I am so glad to have known Ben. I had not really met anyone like him before and I have met few since.

Smiling and welcoming, he had such a genuine excitement and interest in so much of life and a wonderful ability to share that enthusiasm through his commitment and his broad smile. Such an energy for life he had, such imagination, such silliness, such positivity and care, what a wonderful friend, brother, and uncle.

Always smiling and very much part of my youth.

He was a truly lovely human being.

I know that he lived fearlessly and rejoiced in every new day.

I do know that he deserves the wonderful freedom he now has. The rucksack has been cast off and Ben is sitting on the peak of his mountain with a smile on his face. He is surrounded by light, a light we cannot imagine, its beauty is overwhelming.

Then we all gathered together, facing a lovely photo of Ben smiling out at us, while Trustees from Shape East and others—some of them in tears—with whom he had recently been working spoke of his gifts and enthusiasm for the job; his wife, his father, his mother-in-law and other family members spoke of his lovely nature.

And at the end, the mother of his godson leapt to her feet with an exquisite paper parasol Ben had decorated with lines of his poetry, a kind of blessing for the boy's christening many years ago and read it out to us:

> *Let the sun bless your breath,*
> *Let the moon nurture your dreams,*
> *Let the stars sing in your bones,*
> *May this earth nourish your fire.*
> *This water sustain your journey.*
> *Let every tree know your hands,*
> *Let every river know your face,*
> *Let every valley know your feet,*
> *May this sky shelter your mind.*
> *May every rainbow color your smile*
> *And show you the way*

To see your heart is
A Universe of Peace
And each particle within it
A Sacred Happiness.

It was a lovely way to end, but for me the most utterly poignant moment was when, accompanying himself on guitar, his brother-in-law, Luke, sang this song which Ben had written and which Luke had set to music:

I lay down
Down on my heart
'Til morning

Can I find it?
Is it a place?

High up a mountain,
Down by the sea
I'll take this train to the pure land.

I leave the red lights, I leave the grey skies
I leave the billboards, our history.
I leave the car fumes, I leave the hard days
I leave this darkness, and my past lives.

Catch a shooting star (take me back)
A small step as you are (just take me back)
A sunflower's in your heart (please take me back)
This is where I start.

I wake up early; I wake up on the ground.
I see a blue sky, I feel it all around.
I hear a bell sing, at sunrise,
I feel a smile grow.

I have arrived.

I lay down
Down on my heart
'Til morning

Can I find it?
Is it a place?

High up a mountain
Down by the sea
I'll take this train to the pure land.

"Did he perhaps have a premonition?" a friend of Ben and Vicky's asked me afterwards. I don't know whether she had had this thought because of the song she had just heard, but she had in fact voiced a question that had been with me somewhere distant ever since he died: somewhere distant which had come to the fore when I heard the question in the Sunflower Song: "*Can I find it? Is it a place? I'll take this train to the pure land . . .*" Yes, the Pure Land: the Buddhists "other shore";[1] the realm of no "thing-ness" where all has been let go: now *that* surely is Nirvana: the ultimate letting go toward which he seems to have been almost knowingly moving:

> *I leave the red lights, I leave the grey skies,*
> *I leave the billboards, our history.*
> *I leave the car fumes, I leave the hard days*
> *I leave this darkness and my past lives . . .*

And later, "*Take me back; just take me back. This is where I start: I wake up early. I wake up on the ground, I see a blue sky, I feel it all around. I hear*

---

1 "Listen to the Mantra, the Great, Mysterious Mantra: *Gate, gate, paragate, parasam-gate, bodhi, svaha!* Gone, gone, gone to that other shore, safely passed to that other shore, O Prajna-paramita! So may it be." (from the Maha-prajna-paramita sutra)

a bell sing, at sunrise I feel a smile grow. I have arrived . . . " Is it longing I hear? Understanding? Acceptance? Did he come early—because of his frequent illness—to face the fact that we will all die? Was he able to live often with the grave injunction to remember this fact—injunction which is to be found in many sacred writings ancient and modern?

And then, nearly a year after the celebration, I came across this extraordinary piece he had written when he was 19:

Confidential Shame
Black.
Everyone was wearing black.
One of them had a purple tie.
A wreath of red roses protecting the coffin.
My mother was shedding tears, attempts to hold them back in vain; and my sister was sniffling with my grandmother.
We all paced out of the door into the bitter graveyard.
Somebody was going to read. His voice was drained in the bitter breeze. His lips jolted me. I noticed it was a poem my brother had written for a homework. I had helped him with it. My breath was jumping. My eyes blurring.
Focus.
I tightened my nostrils, closed my mouth and breathed in.
My jawbone relaxed and I was crying too.
Sorrow.
He had read it nothing like my brother had meant it to be read. That annoyed me.
That fact, this fact, the fact that he was dead had not yet penetrated my mind. This made me cry, too much.
It was all so cold and slow.
It hurt, something inside my heart, lungs, stomach hurt.
My stomach muscles tightened and my heart ascended to my throat.
The stone floor was colder than cold.
Bitter.
All sounds were not received. I sniffed once more as a tear slid down the crevice of my nose.

Precise steps of the undertakers carrying, a gift, for the ground?
A gift of death.
Will he die? Is he dead?
Who will answer?
Confidential shame.

Will he die? Is he dead? Who will answer?

I will answer Yes, he died. He is not dead.

Chapter 7

Muslim Cab Driver I

Three days before this celebration of Ben's life: 12 October 2006. I take a minicab to have tea with a faithful Austrian friend, who happens to be in London. He had known Ben and will be with us in Cambridge.

As we are driving down Park Lane, the cab driver asks me if I am having a good day? Is it, I wonder, because I have dressed up a bit, as later I will be going on to celebrate the 90th birthday of another special friend—the "Bernard" spoke of so lovingly at the height of his last illness.

"Yes and no," I tell him. I am still in that place where I need to, have to tell anyone who will listen about Ben. "I am going to see a very good friend from overseas . . . but . . . my son died and . . . "

The driver interrupts, "Oh!" he cries, from the heart. "That is the worst thing . . . for a mother . . . the worst thing." And tells me the sad tale of the death in childhood of a brother and how their parents never recovered from this blow.

As I get out of the cab he says. "Pray to Allah . . . You must pray to Allah for Allah always listens to the prayers of the mother . . . And I will pray too . . . "

Muslim Cab Driver II

December 2007 and another minicab ride across town with a driver from Bangladesh.

I have hardly put on my seat belt before he bursts out, "My son died ... 28 years old ... four months ago ... of normal [sic] causes ... normal causes ... My only son ... three daughters ... my only son ... and inside I am burning, burning ... I cannot weep ... I show nothing, but inside I am exploding ... everything has changed ... nothing worth living for, but I make sure my family are all right ... but for me ... it is the end ... pointless ... "

When he finally pauses in his devastated flow I say: "You won't believe this, but this has just happened to me ... " and I tell him about Ben.

I tell him how for weeks afterwards my stomach was filled with churning sensations as if a million butterflies were living there.

"Yes, yes, I know that!" he cries. "That is what it is like for me ... but I cannot weep. My wife weeps all the time, but I cannot ... "

"Are you religious?" I ask him cautiously.

"Yes," he replies almost impatiently, as if it must be obvious. "I am Muslim".

"Does it help you?"

"Yes, for a time. Every morning I get up and wash ... and I pray ... and for a time I am calmer, quieter, but it does not last ... but if I did not pray it would be worse ...

We have to believe in fate ... what is to be, will be ... it was his time ... his time to go from here ... "

"We are living in a world here in the West where we try to pretend death doesn't exist ... "

"Yes. Yes. But that is not good. In my religion we are told to remember forty times a day that we will die ... There is a story that the Angel of Death holds his trumpet in one hand and in the other he holds food, but he never dares put it to his mouth, to eat it, in case at that very moment Allah calls upon him to blow his trumpet for someone's death ... "

We part warmly, bound outside our many seeming differences by the universality of our sorrow ... parents who have outlived their children, looking out at a world with a completely changed vision ...

Chapter 8

The Help of Friends

When Ben died I had a desperate need to communicate, to tell people what had happened. And the response from many of our friends was immediate and sensitive, seeming able to pick up from what I said the essential words which gave away what was preoccupying me.

Help of a very high quality came to me, mostly from our many lifelong steadfast American friends.

First, about a week after the funeral, I received a text from one of them,[1] quoting A. K. Coomaraswamy:[2]

> *If all the preparations have been made correctly, the arrow, like a homing bird, will find its own goal; just as the man who, when he departs from this world "all in act" having done what there was to be done, need not wonder what will become of him, nor where he is going, but will inevitably find the bull's eye, and passing through the sun door, enter into the empyrean beyond the "murity" of the sky.*

A difficult writer, Coomaraswamy, often, one feels, rather like Krishnamurti, irritated and impatient with his readers for not being able to

---

1   Roger Lipsey, who 30 years ago edited two magnificent volumes of Coomaraswamy's essays on Metaphysics and Sacred Art.

2   One time Curator of Oriental Art at the Boston Museum of Fine Art, an exceptional scholar and polymath with a profound spiritual insight.

keep up with him and his insistence on meticulous precision in order of thought and choice of words, but for this very reason these words pierced my heart like the arrow of which he speaks. And I assume he "invented" the word "murity" to signify the "wallness" of the sky which has to be penetrated for the man who "having done what there was to be done" to pass into an immensity and a mystery of which I certainly can have no knowledge.

Mystery . . .

How lightly I have bandied this word about and how lightly I hear now others do so . . . with what banal conviction that I know nevertheless what it is . . .

I only understand the levity now Ben is dead and I am obliged to stand in front finally of mystery. Where is he? *I want to KNOW.* How is he? *I want to know.*

I can't know. The one thing I *do* know at times is that I am using, am obliged to use, a language which is a non-sense in relation to what cannot be known, here, seeing as we do "through a glass, darkly."

The stark etymology of mystery has to do with the notion of standing silent in front of the unknown.

And I quickly see how I am using the only tools I seem to have— words, to try to speak of the unspeakable. Everything spoken of in linear terms, time terms . . .

I can't know from that place . . .

Can I know from *any* place?

———

Closely following Coomaraswamy's arrow came a very timely and also very similar reminder of the depth of wisdom in the Upanishads, when another dear friend in America sent me the following:

> When a person goes forth from this world, he comes to
> the air. It opens out there for him like the hole of a chariot
> wheel. Through that he goes upwards. He goes to the sun.
> It opens out there for him like the hole of a large drum.

> *Through that he goes upwards. He reaches the moon. It*
> *opens out there for him like the hole of a small drum.*
> *Through that he goes upwards. He comes to a world free*
> *from grief, where there are no extremes of heat and cold,*
> *without snow. There he dwells for eternal years.*

And then one of many from the same source, affecting me powerfully because it spoke of the heart and of light; poignant as we knew by then that Ben's heart was undergoing examination at Papworth Hospital; affecting because with him particularly I had always turned to imagery of light, instinctively feeling that light has all to do with love and healing:

> *The point of his heart becomes lighted up, and by that*
> *light the self departs, either through the eye or through*
> *the head, or through other apertures of the body. And*
> *when he thus departs, life departs after him. And when*
> *life thus departs, all the vital breaths depart after him.*
> *He becomes one with intelligence. What has intelligence*
> *departs with him. His knowledge and his work take hold*
> *of him as also his past experience.*

No, not ordinary mind's store of knowledge and no, not going to the office daily. This knowledge as *gnosis*, as direct experience innerly of other levels, other meaning; this work, the interior and accumulated efforts at "present moment, wonderful moment" as Thich Nhat Hanh, Ben's spiritual example, says.

Thanks to this reminder, I too turned to the Upanishads which, although I had studied them quite deeply long ago, I had not thought of for myself. And found there again and again light and the heart to be at the center of their extraordinary, visionary way with words to try to convey the subtleties which lie, like another body, within the physical body, and which do not, cannot perish when we die mortally.

Page after page, scattered through nearly all of them, particularly in the Brihadaranyaka Upanishad and the Chandogya Upanishad, came bone-clean insight. I say bone-clean, imagining the skeleton white and free of all cover-up, just itself . . . No decorations, no poesy, something paramount, pure, pared down to the essential . . . .

"The person made of mind, the light, the true, is inside the heart, like a rice-grain or a barleycorn. He is the ruler of everything, the overlord of everything: he controls all this, whatever there is."[1]

> Janaka, the King of Bihar, came down quietly from his throne and said: "Homage to you, Yajnavalkya: Teach me!"
>
> He said: "King! As one about to make a long journey is furnished with ship or carriage, so you have a self well prepared for the Upanishads, these inner teachings. You have studied the Vedas and the Upanishads, these inner teachings; where will you go, when you leave this world?"
>
> Janaka said: "Blessed one, I do not know where I shall go."
>
> Yajnavalkya said: "Then I will tell you where you will go."
>
> Janaka said: "Tell me, blessed one."
>
> Yajnavalkya said: "In the right eye Self lives and kindles the light; in the left eye His queen. The place where they meet in praise together is the hollow of the heart, their food is the heart's red lump, and their garment is the mesh-like substance of veins within the heart. The path along which they travel is the artery, the channel that goes upward from the heart. The veins established rooted in the heart are as fine as a hair split a thousandfold.
>
> Through the heart flows a food finer than the food that nourishes the body."

How these words, thousands of years old, brought some comfort to

---

1 Brihadaranyaka Upanishad V:6

this mother. There was gratitude, but as well as gratitude, a trust, that I was clearly far, far from alone in experiencing intimations of another life within the planetary life, a coming and going between form and formlessness, perhaps those very "intimations of immortality" of which Wordsworth wrote in his greatest poem.[1] Not, though, of a kind of eternal life, a future life, but another kind of life? Or a return to the source, from which we come "trailing clouds of glory," a return to the source, a finding of our "original face"; the face we had before we were born. Ben, I told myself, had gone back, not on. For some reason this was important to me, the feeling he had gone back, not on . . .

> East, west, north, south, above, below, every quarter is filled with the Self's breath. That Self, described as "not this, not that," is undecaying, for he is not subject to decay. He has nothing sticking to him, for he does not stick to anything. He cannot be grasped, nor destroyed, nor captured, nor afflicted, does not come to harm. That Self is imperishable. Do not fear.[2]

> In this body, in this town of Spirit, there is a little house

---

1 Our birth is but a sleep and a forgetting; The Soul that rises with us, our life's Star/, Hath had elsewhere its setting/And cometh from afar/O joy! That in our embers/ Is something that doth live;/That Nature yet remembers/What was so fugitive!... those obstinate questionings of sense and outward things,/Fallings from us, vanishings;/Blank misgivings of a creature/Moving about in worlds not realized./High instincts, before which our mortal nature /Did tremble like a guilty thing surprised/... those shadowy recollections,/Which be they what they may,/Are yet the fountain-light of all our day,/Are yet a master-light of all our seeing;/Uphold us, cherish, and have power to make/Our noisy years seem moments in the being/Of the eternal Silence: truths that awake,/To perish never;/Which neither listlessness, nor mad endeavor,/Nor man, nor boy/Nor all that is at enmity with joy,/Can utterly abolish or destroy!/Hence, in a season of calm weather/Though inland far we be,/Our souls have sight of that immortal sea/Which brought us hither;/Can in a moment travel thither/And see the children sport upon the shore,/ And hear the mighty waters rolling evermore. —from *Ode on Intimations of Immortality From Recollections of Early Childhood*

2 Brihadaranyaka Upanishad IV:2

shaped like a lotus, and in that house there is a little
space. One should know what is there. What is there?
Why is it so important?

There is as much in that little space within the heart, as there is in the
whole world outside. Heaven, earth, fire, wind, sun, moon, lightning,
stars; whatever is, and whatever is not, everything is there.
If everything is in man's body, every being, every de-
sire, what remains . . . when the body falls? What lies in
that space, does not decay when the body decays, nor does
it fall when the body falls. That space is the home of Spirit
. . . Self is there, beyond decay and death . . .[1]

Again and again as the months go by I return here to sublime insight,
free of all sentimentality; lofty, no "dumbing down."

And when my inner state is sufficiently affected and aided by all
this *gnosis*, this *prajna*, this wisdom, this "in-wit," I remember a brief
exchange long ago with the pupil of Gurdjieff's I most loved, most re-
spected. After listening to him speaking in a vein very much akin to
what I have been quoting and reflecting upon above, I suddenly heard
my self, my little self cry out with a kind of petty indignation: "But how
do you know all this?" To which he replied with a quiet authority, quite
definitely not coming from *his* little self: "*I* know."

Well, thirty years later, when I am in touch with this higher level, I too
can say I know.

But the contact does not last. It cannot last. It is not meant to last . . .
"Loftiness" can suddenly seem far, far away from my subjective sorrow.

I continue to be astonished, taken by surprise, by how quickly my
state can change from relative equanimity in front of this great loss—
that state where I am closer to the higher nature, to the I-AMness which
has always been there—to a state of utter desolation, anguish, despair,
deep, deep grief.

---

1   Chandogya Upanishad 8:1

But what of *Ben's* suffering? For he suffered terribly. I have to face this fact. It was not sublime, it was not bliss, it was not lofty. It was hell.[1] Long periods of malaise, followed by numerous bouts of acute illness: every decade of his life was marked by serious illness. And then from January 2005 until his death in July 2006 ever-increasing sickness; frequent episodes of prolonged vomiting, prolonged hiccoughing; total exhaustion; unpleasant internal examinations; ever increasing medication; major surgery twice; diagnosis of cancer; a cardiac arrest which put him into a medically induced coma for nearly three days; burns on his arm; clots in his arm (from the CPR); nine months chemotherapy, with a second drug added in barely two months before he died; nausea; peripheral neuropathy; gross fatigue; dry, cracking skin on hands; eyelashes falling out; eyebrows falling out; and in the last weeks excruciatingly painful mouth ulcers....

JOB—how could I not think of him? This seemingly shared fact and experience—that through an onslaught on the physical body can come a very great insight and understanding and love of something "far finer than the food that nourishes the physical body." How else to explain the radiance, the love, the joy in life, the delight in the simplest pleasures that shone out almost all of the time from his smiling face, from his very being? ("Yet in my flesh shall I see God..."[2])

And then, months after his death, agonizing over his suffering, but also amazed at how his being shone valiantly through it all, I turn a page in the Brihadaranyaka Upanishad only to find:

"When one suffers from illness, that is the highest asceticism. To suffer from a sickness is surely the highest austerity. Whoever knows

---

1 Yet just once—just once the answer-phone caught the depths of his despair in his voice, almost unrecognizable, heavy, heavy and low and thick with physical and emotional suffering: I hear it now: "Hello, Mum. Ben here."

2 The Book of Job, 19:26

this wins the highest world." (With, in one version, a little note: "This chapter suggests that the most unwelcome experiences can be used for spiritual training.")

I am then also reminded of the appalling and lengthy suffering of William Segal,[1] another good friend, after a car accident which should have killed him. As he lay in hospital after the umpteenth surgery to restore his shattered face and limbs, he was visited by a Japanese friend, abbot of a Zen monastery, who said to him, "Lucky man. One accident like yours is worth 10,000 sittings in a monastery."[2]

In the same, autobiographical part of the book, William Segal says of that terrible time:

"All people who go through a serious illness probably come close to a transformation . . . One is never quite the same. Serious illness must be like a mini-death, at least a foretaste of death. Everything changes."

To read these simple words written in our time not only confirms for me what I find in the Upanishads, but, if I dare say it, almost eclipse them, or at least bring closer to me than ever the conviction that this was indeed Ben's experience.

And when I read in *The Tibetan Book of the Dead* and other Tibetan Buddhist writings that as death approaches all negative emotions vanish, I recall immediately that I was not the only one close to him who witnessed that disappearance in Ben in the last few months, weeks, days of his life.

From the very beginning of his illness in January 2005, I had daily tried to "pray" for my son. I would find a quiet moment, a quiet room, take the phone off the hook and sitting down for a while I would try to visualize him, picture him from the top of his head to the tips of his toes. Drawing on my knowledge and simple practice of Buddhist ways I would imagine that great light was shining down upon him above his

---

1 Business man, artist, writer and pupil of G. I. Gurdjieff.
2 Quoted by Marielle Bancou-Segal in *A Voice at the Borders of Silence*.

head, and pouring through him, as if to bring strength and a healing energy. I had long ago taught myself the Tibetan Buddhist *Vajrasattva*, the "One Hundred Syllable Mantra" which is used for healing, which must never be confused with curing. Following this teaching, and reciting the Sanskrit syllables out loud, but quietly, I would visualize, just above the head, the union of active and passive energies in the form of a male and a female conjoined, making this energy and allowing it to flow into him as if to purify him and give him strength.

(As I write this it has suddenly come back to me that I tried this on the morning after his surgery on 14 July 2005. When I visited him later that same day he told me that suddenly in the middle of the morning he had felt as if all the bad things in his body had been taken out and away and he had been filled with a good, positive, heartening feeling.)

It seems to me that whatever is tried out of total love for another's deep, real need, has some kind of effect beyond our understanding. And the reciting of syllables in an unknown language, at the very least, makes it impossible for the mind to be distracted by personal demand, (a wrong sort of prayer expecting insisting on a result) ego, associations, unhelpful emotions such as fear or anxiety.

However, I very soon discovered that I could not by any means always rise to the heights of all these wisdoms, but I could at least visualize Ben as surrounded with light and the mother-love, "immeasurable, immutable."

As I bent over him when he was coming out of his medically induced coma, kissing him on his cold, cold forehead gently, so, so gently, I murmured "Love. Light."

And he nodded.

As I bent over to kiss his cold, cold forehead in the hospital chapel the day after he died, I murmured, "Love, darling. Love . . . Light . . . "

And when now I sit in meditation or prayer I seem to see him facing me cross-legged and again I visualize that golden light pouring down upon him, and rainbow light surrounding him, the glorious colors that belong to the five meditation buddhas[1] lighting him on his way, surely, to some "pure land"—

It was months before I found any words in the Christian gospels which spoke to me and then suddenly I heard: "In my father's house are many mansions. If it were not so I would have told you. I go to prepare a place for you . . ."[2]

And realized Christ was speaking of dimensions—that there are other dimensions, there must be other dimensions. The second sentence suggests that He could be trusted. I also later wondered if the third sentence was telling us that He was perhaps talking not only of the imminent physical death, and a departure in temporal language to another place—"Heaven"?—but was speaking of another kind of prepared place, prepared by example. A place within? Elsewhere, in material some bishops long, long ago decided should be omitted from the Four Gospels, a disciple describes a vision afforded to him at the very moment in time when Christ was on the cross, saying: "I held fast this one thing in myself, that the Lord contrived all things symbolically and by a dispensation toward men, for their conversion and salvation."[3] And I assume that in speaking of "conversion" he does not mean what that has come to mean, but rather that *metanoia*, that "turning around in the seat of consciousness" which is spoken of in the Buddhist Lankavatara Sutra.

Then one day I suddenly heard those powerful words, until now not understood:

"Verily, verily I say unto you: Before Abraham was, I AM."[4]

---

1 Each with his own complete transformative qualities; his own "radiant light," blue, yellow, red, green, white; each related to a specific element, a specific wisdom; his own sacred sound; his own sacred gesture.

2 St John's Gospel, 14:2

3 Apocryphal New Testament, Acts of John 102

4 St John's Gospel, 8:58

And it came to me that they might mean that that part in us, that inner-most part, at the heart's center, IS ALWAYS—beyond the time world of man, however far back we care to go. This I AM exists outside all the laws we convince ourselves much of the time govern our lives . . .

"*Before Abraham was, I AM.*"

As I absorbed the uplifting energy in these words I remembered, as I had so often during the last years of Ben's life, how when aged 16 he underwent drastic, life-saving surgery, Henri Tracol phoned me from the south of France to ask after him and simply said: "I am with you." I remembered too that I had at once understood that he did not mean himself, his little *persona*, but himself as representative of this immense, immortal I AM. I found myself able to lean once more into those pow-erful little words.

"*Before Abraham was, I AM.*"

Not for the first time I was struck by the simple and brief way in which Christ always states the essential kernel of His inspiring vision—like all great teachers and visionaries—the more important the vision the shorter the number of words, the fewer the syllables. Many great poets and mystics from across the centuries come to mind here:

"Thy will be done in[1] earth as it is in heaven . . . Give us this day our daily bread . . . "

> *And all shall be well*
> *And all manner of thing shall be well.*

> —Julian of Norwich

> *Teach me my God and king in all things thee to see*
> *And what I do in any thing,*
> *To do it as for thee.*

> —George Herbert

---

1   It is interesting and sad to note that at some point the "in earth" of *The Book of Com-mon Prayer* which surely refers to the "planetary" body was changed to "*on* earth."

You must go through the way in which you are not.
And what you do not know is the only thing you know
And what you own is what you do not own
And where you are is where you are not.

—T. S. Eliot

And of course from Shakespeare, I could cover page after page of examples:

Speak what we feel, not what we ought to say.

The readiness is all.

Full fathom five thy father lies;
Of his bones are coral made:
Those are pearls that were his eyes:
Nothing of him that doth fade,
But doth suffer a sea change
Into something rich and strange . . .

And now I hear myself saying: Full fathom five my son now lies. Nothing of him that doth fade . . . but doth suffer a change into something rich and strange.

—

Another friend sent me the words of Mother Maria of Paris (1891–1945), a Russian Orthodox saint of our times, and who perished in Ravensbruck, written when *her* child died:

Into the black, yawning grave fly all hopes, plans, hab-
its, calculations, and—above all—meaning: the mean-
ing of life. Meaning has lost its meaning, and another
incomprehensible Meaning has caused wings to grow
at one's back . . . and I think that anyone who has had

> *this experience of eternity, if only once; who has under-*
> *stood the way he is going, if only once; who has seen the*
> *One who goes before him, if only once—such a person*
> *will find it hard to turn aside from the path: to him all*
> *comfort will seem ephemeral, all treasures valueless, all*
> *companions unnecessary, if among them he fails to see the*
> *One companion carrying his Cross.*

If I consider "the One" as the "I AM" deep within me, the "I" who knows, then I can say I have met that One more than once.

If I consider Christ as the incarnation, the embodiment of that One, then I feel at one with the tradition I was raised in, steeped in, well into early adulthood when I began to discover *that* One was far from alone in calling my attention to that "I AM" secretly dwelling within me, as it does, but most of the time unattended, in every one of us.

Only now, and only sometimes, but then most surely, I know that the more his illness seemed to be consuming Ben's physical "planetary" body, as Gurdjieff called it, the more I tried to be there with him, to meet him as he was shedding the skins, the layers of planetary life, the more often we were granted to connect with each other from those secret places within us both.

———

From the onset of Ben's last illness, in January 2005, I was drawn, without really understanding why, to the wisdom of Tibetan Buddhism. With their powerful sacred texts, particularly what we in the West know as *The Tibetan Book of the Dead* (but which is known to the Tibetans as *The Great Liberation on Hearing*), and which I have been studying on and off for over thirty years, they seem to *know* what happens at death in a way which I have not yet found in any other sacred teaching. Familiar with 3 or 4 different translations, and having read and re-read several learned attempts to "explain" its meaning, I returned once more to this material, appreciating more than ever the insistence that this teaching is intended to be studied and practiced all through life and not merely at the moment of death. In it we are told that life, dying, the after death state, and rebirth consist of a number of bardos or gaps, or spaces "in-between," within the "nowness" of which, if we are present to that, a change of direction becomes possible toward liberation from having to come back "down" here again into *samsara*, this ever-turning wheel of existence.

The first *bardo* is the time between being born and dying, the state we know best, of waking and sleeping in the ordinary sense.

The second bardo, also experienced during this period between birth and death, is the dream state we enter into every night.

The third bardo is the state experienced during meditation and which is the great help available to us throughout life as preparation for death.

The fourth bardo is the "painful bardo" of dying, during which the dissolution and disintegration of the body is experienced in defined stages.

The fifth bardo is the state experienced immediately on the realization that one is physically dead, that one has left the physical body.

At the moment of death a great clear light appears, all negativity vanishes and if aware of this extraordinary moment one is released from rebirths altogether and enters either a "pure land" or even *nirvana*—a state of "no-thing-ness," of no more "coming or going," nor more being born, dying and being born again into the wheel of existence. However, unless one has prepared for death during life one will fall unconscious at that moment and move on to the sixth bardo where one will be drawn irrevocably toward a new birth, a new round of existence.

As I write this it comes to me directly, and not as an idea, that I have "to be there" if there is to be any change of direction, and that I have to practice this being here now and often for the rest of my "of the earth, earthy" life.

Yes, but also as I write this I ask what of sudden death? What then? And am still seeking for an answer somewhere among the sacred traditions.

Chapter 9

Orientation

Disorientation. Or a new orientation?

Shock.

Disorientation.

I have been undone by this death.

Come to a halt.

Quite unable to turn within.

Full of questions as to what I understand.

Acknowledgment of the truth of mystery.

What has happened is indeed a mystery.

And I don't want it to be. I don't want to accept mystery—that word—
that word which the dictionary defines as "anything kept concealed or
very obscure"; "that which is beyond human knowledge to explain"
from the Greek *mysterion-mystes*; and etymology gives as coming from
the Greek root "to close the eyes; suggested by the Greek 'mu', a slight
sound with closed lips"; and in all the definitions a hint of the need to
be initiated into mystery.

I thought this, said this, wrote this more than once in the first months after Ben's death.

But there came a day in March 2007 when I felt, at last, that I could welcome the fact of mystery. I was happy, relieved, glad even, that there is mystery, which leads to awe, defined in the dictionary as "a reverential wonder or fear"—fear, I trust, in the sense of something far, far beyond my comprehension, my puny human comprehension.

And stemming from this new perception, this new experience, disorientation *turned* into a new orientation, given direction by those words of Christ: *Before Abraham was, I AM.*

Chapter 10

Zombie

I am a zombie—at times I am a zombie.

An automaton.

I see myself going through the motions, functioning mostly quite well—and when I do see this I try to hone my attention—preparing food, cooking, washing up, tidying, shopping, etc.

I hear myself speaking—as if I were not the one speaking. What voice, whose voice is coming out of my mouth? Who is this person? Is this me?

Hollow, hollow, hollow. Empty sounds but which seem to perfectly satisfy the hearer. The hearer does not seem to hear or see it is a zombie speaking, a zombie stacking the dishes, arranging flowers, emptying compost . . .

Chapter 11

Dreams

I long for them. I long for him to come to me in a dream, in dreams, but it has not happened . . . yet.

The nearest I have come to dreaming of him—Ben a little blonde boy, perhaps four years old, coming up the front path and somehow arriving with me in our back garden. We are near the steps to the house. His father and his sisters are in the distance, in the garden itself. I tell his father, "Come quickly. He isn't going to be here for very long."
    End of dream.
    Quite soon after he died I had lots of dreams where he was not . . . and yet somehow they were about him. Conspicuous by his very absence. Crowds of people as if on the periphery of a great big HOLE . . .
    Or I would dream that some friend or other was asking me, "What happened?" And I would be telling them . . .

Strange that I have not dreamt about him, since I have had in the past some very vivid dreams about dear ones who have died. I would almost not call them "dreams" but "visitations"—

———

Why doesn't he come? I comfort myself by thinking perhaps it is because he is so close, in flesh and blood and marrow-bone, there is no "need."
    Or am I not recognizing the way in which he comes?

Sometimes when I am sitting in the Buddhist sense, I hear "Mum" ... and I say "Ben" and he says "Mum."

Once I sensed light piercing me through the center of my head down into my forehead and again his "voice."

I talk to him, of course. Mostly to say "sorry, darling" when I have negative thoughts, bitter thoughts. "Sorry, darling, for bringing my darkness anywhere near you ... "

"Sorry, darling, if my weeping makes it dark around you ... "

Chapter 12

Postcard

I find the postcard of a Matisse paper-cut from Ben, December 2002, written to us when a very dearly loved family friend died.

And in it he answers my now so often repeated question: Where are you?

"I am sure that people of such quality do not really "go" anywhere—they just "change" their form. I am sure she will—and has—become part of you both..."

I ask myself, is the reason he does not "come to me" in dreams because he is already, always has been, part of us both?

Chapter 13

"Lovely Jubbly!"

Once when we were alone together in the year before he died, walking in balmy spring warmth and natural beauty I heard myself say, "Look thy last on all things lovely every hour."

This came back to me this morning, a very mild March day with all the flowers and blossom trees around me . . .

Why I suddenly said that I don't know, but he said, "Gosh! What's that Mum?"

"I think it was from a poem by Robert Bridges, a one time Poet Laureate . . . "

"Did he really say that? Gosh . . . ."

It seems to me now, looking back on the last year or so of his life, that he was always looking his last on all things lovely—every hour . . . .

Of course he had some very bad moments, very bad indeed—of despair, of weeping, let alone of pain, much physical wretchedness and discomfort; but it was amazing how often he managed to rise above them, return so quickly to his good spirits, his love of life, his positive attitude. He had his "lovely girls," his wife, his daughter, who gave him so much joy and raison d'être.

I have lost count of the times he would say to me, "It's all right, Mum, it's just a *thing*, this cancer, this illness, this chemo. It's just a *thing*."

A simple stroll round the gardens near our house, a simple stroll on a cold, dank, grey winter's day, but in the company of his wife, his child, his parents, his sister and her family, would be described later as, "That was a lovely afternoon. I couldn't have been happier, Mum . . . "

"Lovely jubbly . . . "

Chapter 14

Yourself First

Yourself first, or not . . .

Ben had barely recovered from the cardiac arrest in July 2005 before the doctors were "after" him about starting chemotherapy. He was advised to make a decision fairly quickly as the most promising "window" for good results was open for about 2–3 months at most. He took his time; consulted the specialists including the gastroenterologist who had cared for him since the onset of the ulcerative colitis 27 years ago; talked it over with his wife.

Then, the decision made to proceed (he was to tell me later that he decided on that because he knew that if the cancer came back he would never forgive himself for letting Vicky and his child down . . .); the treatments began in October 2005 . . .

Of course I went into a frenzied action of researching what might help him through the chemotherapy.

I bought the Bristol Cancer Care Center's video. We offered to pay for him to go there on whichever of their courses might help him most.

I ordered him regular supplies of the very best multi-vitamin and mineral supplements I could find.

And later when his hands grew dry and stained and cracked from the chemo side-effects I found a wonderful salve which really seemed to help.

I bought a rice steamer in the hope this would help to simplify and speed up the cooking of a staple which he found he enjoyed and could easily digest. I don't think it was ever used; a good juicer which was—every day, often more than once.

Before I sent him the Bristol video I watched it myself. It was full of useful information and advice, the most important being that you must, must, must *put yourself first*.

But he didn't—ever.

It was not in his nature. *He* was the carer, the nurturer, the supporter. He may never have looked it up in the dictionary, but he was the epitome of *devotion*, of giving himself *to*—the ones he loved, loved *unconditionally*, to the work he loved, to the world he loved.

And although he said he really wanted to go to Bristol, deep down in my heart I knew from day one that he would never go. It did not take me long to see and understand that he simply did not have the energy. (He went on working full-time for several months into the 9 month chemo ordeal). But also he could not bear to be parted from his little family; could not entertain the thought of leaving all the care of their child to his hard-pressed wife, who was also working part-time (as well as at home at all hours, often late into the night).

Since his death I have read of cancer sufferers who obeyed the edict—yourself first—to the letter and beyond, so very understandably. Since his death I have spoken with a brave one recently diagnosed with cancer—a wife, a mother, a grandmother, telling me firmly "From now on I am going to put myself first," but knowing that neither she nor I really believed that she really would be able to . . .

I begin to understand something about *love*. And *need*.

It became evident very quickly that help was needed; that he would not ask for it, expect it—indeed to the very end of his life he was always thanking us for what we did. The subject of one of his e-mails even was "gratitude."

Chapter 15

Icon

10 November 2007
I see an icon entitled "Mother, do not weep for me."

The Virgin Mary is leaning toward Christ on the cross.
These words are taken from part of the great Russian Orthodox Easter service.

It is not the "Don't cry, Mummy" of the child who is frightened by the mother's tears, the tears of its All Protector.
It is the cry of the child who perceives deep grief beyond bearing.
It is more even than that here: it is almost a command from the child who has grown far, far beyond the mother in understanding.
Can I hear an echo here for me, from *my* child and lean into it?

Dear mother, dear mother, do not weep for me.
Your weeping does me harm . . .

There's a rose and a rose and a genteel rose
The charm that grows so green.
God will give us grace in every mortal place
For to pray to our heavenly Queen.

—(from a folksong, Underneath the leaves)

"Your weeping does me harm . . . "

Strange, or is it, to find this deep wisdom not only in the injunctions of the Tibetan Buddhists and other spiritual wellsprings—not to distress the newly dead one by our weeping and wailing, but also in this lovely simple song . . .

Chapter 16

ATOMS

Atoms, molecules, particles in one strand of little Jenna's hair, caught in a sunbeam.

We talk of this . . . Ben thin, pale, but joyful, a few days after his return home from major surgery in July 2005, during that brief lull before the cardiac arrest.

"Dissolution, melting . . . "

"Yes, Mum . . . "

Everything to live for—he had everything to live for.

And yet he could say that "Yes."

He knew, he understood what I meant.

This ever-present, inevitable dissolution—

And it was *all right*.

Chapter 17

Easter 2007

Nine months after Ben's death, and I was searching for material to read with some others on Good Friday and turned, not for the first time, to the Apocryphal New Testament and in particular the Acts of John.

There I read, not for the first time, the extraordinary passage which begins with John's account of the disciples dancing with Christ on the Mount of Olives the night before His arrest.

But it was the passage that follows which spoke to me in a new way:

Now answer thou unto my dancing.

Behold thyself in me who speak, and seeing what I do, keep silence about my mysteries.

Thou that dancest, perceive what I do, for thine is this passion of the manhood which I am about to suffer For thou couldst not at all have understood what thou sufferest if I had not been sent unto thee as the word of the Father. Thou that sawest what I suffer sawest me as suffering, and seeing it thou didst not abide, but wert wholly moved, moved to make wise. [Thou hast me as a bed, rest upon me.]

If thou hadst known how to suffer, thou wouldest have been able not to suffer . . .

I have leapt . . . [1]

---

1 Apocryphal New Testament, Acts of John 96

Here I paused in shock, almost in delight, because I had come across this leaping elsewhere in a 3rd-century piece about Christ as a living tree: "To all of you who love me I say: I have leapt and you have leapt with me."

And I knew then that, by analogy, I could say: Ben has leapt and I have leapt with him.

And immediately I was reminded that on the physical, earth plane, Ben had once indeed leapt—across a chasm in the Sierra Nevada while hiking on the John Muir Trail in California—an adventure he had set himself only a few years before his death—an adventure born of a deep love of the natural world and in particular of the glimpses of it he had already had on earlier trips to San Francisco and Marin County. But an adventure also born of a sense he had of challenge, of risk, knowing as he seems to have from early adolescence that life itself *is* risk.

On his return he described so vividly the moment of that leap that my mother-heart was in my mouth, yet able at the same time to rejoice in his act, sensing how profoundly important it had been for him in all ways.

So now I was here on the first Easter after his death with these sacred texts calling me to understand something not on the physical level, and at the same time suddenly remembering his vivid description of leaping quite literally across a perilous gap, and reaching the other side and hearing in his voice a sense of immense satisfaction. And I experienced directly the existence of these two worlds—the physical and the spiritual. How I wish there were some other word to use than this word "spiritual," whose worth and profound meaning diminishes daily before my very eyes.

It might be fresher, better to speak of two *states*—of form and of formlessness.

Or of this visible world and the invisible world of *spiritus, pneuma, ruach*—invisible but of very real substance, which figures so frequently in all the great "spiritual" traditions, the substance which allows another kind of world to exist, and which we can only experience, while living in the flesh, as breath.

And I saw the cross—I saw my cross as the horizontal plane on which I live in the visible world and at the same time as the vertical axis which allows brief access to this other invisible, this formlessness . . .

I saw "my" cross, but then, I read on in Acts of John, and to my joy I found confirmation of this vision . . .

> Thus . . . having danced with us the Lord went forth. And we, as men gone astray or dazed with sleep fled this way and that. I then, when I saw him suffer, (suffering on the cross) did not even abide by his suffering (did not stay there), but fled unto the Mount of Olives, weeping at what had befallen. And when he was crucified on the Friday, at the sixth hour of the day, darkness came upon all the earth. And my Lord, standing in the midst of the cave, and enlightening it, said: John, unto the multitude below in Jerusalem I am being crucified and pierced with lances and reeds, and gall and vinegar is given me to drink. But unto thee I speak, and what I speak, hear thou.
>
> I put it into thy mind to come up into this mountain, that thou mightest hear those things which it behoveth a disciple to hear from his teacher [and a man from his God]
>
> And having thus spoken, he showed me a cross of light set up and about the cross a great multitude . . .

My analogy is these two states of "mind" or "understanding": "down" I am this multitude . . . lost, not unified. "Above" I enter into formlessness, light, a greater vision and have to accept I will now always be moving between the two.

OR actually—having leapt with Ben—and I have leapt with Ben—and flung into a new domain, as he has been, a domain unknown, except that it is transpersonal, I have to sit beneath this "cloud of unknowing." There is no going back any more than there could have been for John once he had this vision . . . no going back.

Till the day I die I have to live this tension between the horizontal and the vertical—if I really love my son.

Chapter 18

Agony

Great dark pit opened up beneath my feet, the worst so far.

For several days every second thought was about Ben, accompanied by a lunge in the solar plexus as if going down too fast in a lift. A great fluttering in the heart.

Agony.

And the "dark" thoughts, the "dark" questions: how long does it take for a body to decompose? Read in the press of a man's body after five months being found "badly decomposed" . . . after five months, for us now it is ten . . .

Bones last forever, don't they?

What must his dear body have looked like by the time the post mortem investigations had been completed? I picture a sort of stitched up patchwork of flesh . . .

No, no, no. A terrible refusal. Started clicking my teeth again, know I am grinding them in my sleep because of the jaw pain in the mornings. Starting rocking again, back and forth like an old Jewish grannie at prayer. Staring into space . . . feel depression could get a hold. Waves of clamminess all over. Sweat trickles from all the hair follicles on my head.

What helps?

One night on the border of sleep, wracked with the "dark" thoughts, suddenly aware of a strong blue light shimmering between my eyes.

This comes about from time to time, has done for many years. I know I can't make it happen.

It is benevolent, beneficent, loving. I know that in Tibetan Buddhism blue is the color of the Medicine Buddha, and is also the color of the element, ether, which contains all the other elements—water, earth, fire and air—ether, that luminous space where Aksobhya dwells, one of the five Buddhas to be visualized during meditation.

In her book, *Luminous Emptiness*, Francesca Fremantle says of this color blue:

> *Blue is a color of mystery and spirituality; it is associated with heaven, and therefore it has always conveyed the ideas of peace, happiness, beauty and perfection.*

But she goes on to warn of its other aspect:

> *The unfathomable depth of blueness can also carry a threat and a sense of fear . . . the fundamental fear of death, the terror of losing the sense of self, that we confront when we look into the face of the element of space.*

It seems that this is a warning that even at the highest level of direct experience (*gnosis, prajna, jnana*), and the most sincere and serious intention, this other aspect is there, too.

Indeed, elsewhere in her book she warns us of the dangers always present on the spiritual path which is "a continual struggle against delusion and egoism."

I know the truth of this in myself already: there are times when I feel I "know" things now that others who haven't been through this experience don't "know."

It is true, but its truth can be quickly tainted and diminished by a sense of superiority.

I have in fact "nowhere to lay my head,"[1] no permanent resting place,

---

1   The foxes have holes, and the birds of the air have nests, but the Son of Man has

no sense of an ending, and at times I long for some sort of ending, but no, if I am to make use of this terrible sorrow—to extend my possibility as a human being, I cannot settle for the "closure" nowadays so often spoken of, demanded even.

And I find myself welcoming the fact of these two aspects to both of which I need to be present for any real understanding to be possible. When the blue light appears it feels as if a hand is coming down to me from above, rather like those ancient frescoes or mosaics showing "the hand of God" reaching down through clouds and rays of light . . .

And a few times I hear as I have before, "Mum," and my answer, "Ben."

Must not forget *Before Abraham was, I AM.*

What helps?

Know I must "rest" from all this each day for a while. I do. I go to sleep every afternoon with a mask over my eyes, hugging my body. Deep sleep often, so different from the nights.

What helps?

I suddenly remember how some Buddhist monks are sent, or used to be sent, into the "charnel" ground, the burying grounds, made to look at corpses in all stages of decay, down to the bare-boned skeleton in order to impress upon them the impermanence of the physical body. But perhaps not only of that?

But also "of impermanence and the continual presence of death in life" to quote Francesca Fremantle again.

Maybe I am not being morbid with my "dark" thoughts, my "dark" questions.

I notice that they actually seem to be leading me to "believing" that it is true that I am not "just" the body. That there is an energy within it

---

nowhere to lay his head.—Gospel of St. Matthew, 8:20

that goes elsewhere at death. I remember holding down a cat for the vet while he put her to sleep, and as the needle plunged through the fur I felt her energy, her life force leave the body so that now it seemed I had my hands on an empty sack.

What helps?

Stillness. Straight but not tense vertical posture. Head neither bowed down, bent, nor tilted upwards. Awareness of breathing without interference—allowing myself to be breathed.

Chapter 19

Grasping

Suddenly see that I am grasping at comprehension . . .

My futile attempt to force the unknown, the unknowable, to be known, is a kind of grasping . . .

Chapter 20

Friday 6 July 2007

Ben died a year ago today.

And now today we are at the Cottage with Vicky and her close family and Robin, one of Ben's dearest friends, who danced at his wedding, and who, when Ben died wrote:

> For the many years that I knew Ben he had the words
> LIFE IS RISK in bold red letters above his desk in his
> room in Rochester Road, words that he lived as he hurtled
> forwards tasting all the world could offer him. I followed
> him on many of his adventures and always marveled at
> his ability to enlighten, inspire and thrill. His postcards
> and handwritten letters were a beautiful constant in a
> world of speed and ephemeral transience. He pursued so
> many things, continually searching and adding sweet lay-
> ers to his immense being, everything he did from the the-
> ater work to the work with children, to the architecture
> was driven by the belief to strive for excellence, beauty
> and to make the world a better place.
>
> I remember the excitement and joy in his voice when
> he told me about Vicky. Ah yes, she was his queen and
> was to give him the greatest gift he had always longed
> for—the sweet jewel that is Jenna. Never was there a
> more deserving father.
>
> Dearest Ben, we shall keep your memory alive in the
> springtime, rejoice in your laughter in the summer, retreat
> to your love in the winter and wonder at your strength in

the autumn. Ben, my true brother, I offer you the only gift
that I can now, and that is to give a protecting veil over
Vicky and Jenna as long as I live . . .
Ben, all that you were, is that I shall Be—
Never Waste a Moment.
Never Stop Asking Questions.
Make the world a better place.
LIFE IS RISK.

It is a glorious day but without the excessive heat of 6 July 2006.

We have all brought flowers.

We go down to the churchyard to the grave, where the day before his father, in pouring rain, had helped the artist stone-carver to fix the headstone into the earth.

It is absolutely beautiful—Purbeck stone, flecked minutely with fossil-shaped markings, glowing, soft, neither white, nor grey, infused with an inner goldenness.

Ben Koralek
1967-2006

And round the edge, a few stars and lines from one of his poems, written when he was 17, and which his sister, Lucy, had read at the funeral:

In smiling at the world, I see life.
In smiling at the world, I remember.

Little Jenna carries a basket of rosebuds, running, running, sure she knows exactly where her father's "special place" is, and when she finds it strokes the stone, leans on it proprietarily.

A print of her little hand has been carved into it just below ground level, concealed behind a piece of green grass turf. Her grandfather lifts out the turf and she sees her little hand and likes that.

Robin has brought with him a lovely Maori cloth, used at the time of mourning and burial. It is covered with stars and birds in gold thread. He covers the headstone with it while we all scatter our many flowers over the grave—lavender, scabious, roses, orchids, lilies. Then Robin removes the cloth and we stand quietly while Vicky reads a poem. Jenna looks a little sleepy, a little sad, in her other grandmother's arms, who then wisely takes her away. We all slowly return to the house and out in the sunshine on the terrace seek—seek what? Refuge? Solace? Normality? Well, we have tea and cakes.

Some have to leave. The rest of us, Robin, Vicky's mother and brother, stay overnight with us. Jenna takes time to settle into sleep. There is some crying and then the sweet voice in the little bedroom just above us singing, *Frère Jacques* . . . word perfect, and in tune. We have a quiet, gentle, reflective supper, a little wine, talking elliptically around general subjects, but which we all know were dear to Ben's heart—education, children . . . what is lacking for their needs . . . what might be done about that?

There is warmth between us, tenderness—an understanding of the fragility of each one of us and an unspoken recognition, that evening, of the equal measure of our different kinds of love for Ben . . .

Chapter 21

Another Way of Saying

A quite unexpected help came to me today on reading in Gurdjieff's *Beelzebub's Tales to His Grandson*, a beautiful and original way of describing the burying of a dead human being as giving the "planetary 'body' to the presence of the planet . . . "

It enhanced for me suddenly the "belief" which comforts me that indeed what belongs to the earth, earthy, is received and welcomed back, hinting that it might even be organic and therefore enriching food[1] . . .

And these thoughts led me back to St. Paul and his letter to the Corinthians,[2] an extraordinary attempt to grapple with the notion of "degrees," of levels . . . where when he is not "hectoring" a little, he makes so clear that each kind of energy has its place[3] and at those moments he is not so far from Gurdjieff's vision of an "exchange of substances"[4] or Shakespeare's "sea change into something rich and strange."[5]

---

1 To my delight some time later I saw a "nature" film which bore out the fact of this: sometimes salmon leaping up the falls in Alaska flip themselves onto dry land and die. By means of speeded up photography we were shown the gradual disintegration of the fish drawn back into the earth and told that the elements of their flesh and bones are known to feed and enrich the earth.

2 I Corinthian, 15

3 Ibid vv 39-53

4 In *Beelzebub's Tales to His Grandson,* ch. 17

5 In *The Tempest,* act 1, scene 2

Chapter 22

"It" is Not Separate

In the sittings at a retreat recently had a very strong experience of a light coming down in an arrow shape, piercing through center of my forehead, through "third eye"—about as far as top half of face and a sense that I was communicating with Ben.

I know I wasn't literally—well I suppose I wasn't, but I "heard" "Mum" and I "said" "Ben," and it was as if something very fine was opened to this great benevolence which I do know pours down on us all the time.

Something has "happened" to me. I am not speaking in tongues exactly, but words, insights, perceptions are coming through me in a quite different way from before Ben died;[1] although, if I think back, I remember times when something like this was happening during the last two years of his life . . .

---

1 Could I be approaching that stage Hermann Hesse ascribes to the protagonist in *The Journey to the East*: "His suffering became too great and you know that as soon as suffering becomes acute enough one goes forward."

Chapter 23

Someone is Missing

For over a year, whenever the family is gathered all together at our cottage, I feel someone is missing . . .

But at any moment . . . will come round the corner through the rose arch onto the terrace . . .

Or, laying the table . . . how many are we? Seven, eight, nine? Surely there is someone missing . . .

And I cannot get used to just saying, "The girls . . . , " or when people ask how many children do we have, hear myself strangely saying, "We have two daughters and a son who died . . . "

Or if one of the girls asks me how the other one is I am waiting to hear "and Ben?"

He is missing, always, always missing . . .

Chapter 24

Euripides

*"Sweet... always... never... precious... darling... always... never... love
... precious... Always... darling... "*

This is how I remember the broken words in the speech of Andromache
in Katie Mitchell's production of *Women of Troy* after *The Trojan Women*
of Euripides ... when her baby is torn from her and taken away to be
dropped from the battlements and smashed to death ...

In this version of the play the mother walks, glides slowly, slowly
across the stage robed in white and visibly pregnant. Her broken words
and all that lies in sentences behind each one rang completely true to
this grieving mother. The only word missing was "beloved": the only
error, earlier in the play, when, after her daughter is dragged away to
become the "kept woman" of Agamemnon, Hecuba falls down onto her
back, where instinctively I was having her fling herself onto her *belly* in
a completely uncontrollable fall to close contact with Mother Earth, I
suppose ... I just know that that is the natural inclination in all-out
sorrow—to fall *down* and *onto* or into or against something steadier,
stronger, firmer which I can *sink* into, *lean* into, which will *hold* me ...
the floor, the garden grass, the earth, the solid frame of another human
being ...

The broken mother's broken words about her broken son brought me
to tears and yet, on leaving the theater, I realized I was up to a point
experiencing the intended *catharsis*—along with a powerful realization
that there really is "nothing new under the sun," the universality and

endlessness of mothers breaking over the death of a child. The play was written in 415 BCE.

And Hecuba unfolding from a little bag her murdered daughter, Polyxena's clothes slowly, and drawing out the shoes . . . the shoes . . . the shoes . . .

Chapter 25

"Magical Thinking?"

Yes, I know about Joan Didion keeping her dead husband's shoes . . .
just in case . . . as she tells us in *A Year of Magical Thinking*, her austere,
courageous account of *his* sudden death.

Ben's slippers are under the coat stand in the hall . . . and I had not exactly forgotten this, rather pushed it far away at the very back of my mind.

But only a day or two after I had written the above impatiently—
she's not the only one . . . I *know* too, the weather turned suddenly bitterly cold and I went looking for my winter boots, thinking I had left
them from last year underneath that coat-stand. Groping about for
them I put my hand on Ben's slippers . . .

And yes, then I really could say, "I know about Joan Didion and her
husband's shoes . . . "

I pulled out the dust-covered slippers and burst into burning tears . . .
awful.

Trying to "pull myself together," I started brushing the thick dust off
without success. "Don't be silly, "I told myself. "Clean them up and give
them to Oxfam. That's what Ben would want—that they would be of
some use to someone else . . . "

Staring at them, clutching at them, I then heard myself say, "No,
throw them away! Throw them away!"

I even found a plastic bag to put them in to go in the bin.

But I couldn't do it.

I pulled on my winter boots, coat, hat and went out into the little
park where we so often walked with Ben to the playground to put Jenna

on the swings . . . Glorious day . . . pure blue sky; sun; golden plane trees . . . I walked round and round and round, tears still pouring . . .

Came home, took the slippers out of the bag and put into the washing machine. They will go to Oxfam, but it was to be a very long time before I actually took them there . . .

Chapter 26

Crucible

Yes, am in the crucible . . .

Yesterday found some of Ben's throwaway razors and aftershave lotion in the little-used shower-room cupboard at top of house.

In a tearful sobbing blur I collected them all up dumped them into a waste paper basket and emptied them into the rubbish bin outside . . .

Like finding his slippers it provoked a real setback—stabbing pain of the reality of his physical absence . . .

Today, while sitting and having prayed for help, experiencing some degree of my formlessness, I opened to him in his formlessness saying I am with you, always with you, wherever, whatever, and remembering the friend who said he had felt I had always been with Ben "every step of the way," realized I can be and am often still with him every step of the way and suddenly I was back in that shower-room.

Anguish . . . feeling bereft to my very depths, joined momentarily with this other experience of feeling that I am still with him every step of the way and that I am in this crucible of experiences, this necessary blending, this necessary suffering—can it bring about some degree of "change" in me, of—dare I use such a high word—of "transforming" me?

Got up from sitting feeling this churning, this narrowing of the "gyre"[1] . . . Something is "a-stirring" in me, something is "a-transforming" in me . . .

Not done by me. The only thing done by me is the necessary movement to opening in silence, stillness, praying for help, which as Henri once said, "I know is there, for sure" . . .

---

1 This word surfaced from the depths, coated with my understanding of its meaning as a spiral, based on Yeats's use of it in *The Second Coming*:

> Turning and turning in the widening gyre
> The falcon cannot hear the falconer.
> Things fall apart; the center cannot hold.

But where he uses it to express his concern at its widening, making it impossible for the "center to hold," I am trying to use it to express the opposite—a narrowing of the spiral "cone" which would allow the center to hold. And suddenly a striking photo of Ben comes to mind where he stands firm, fearless, strong, arm outstretched, hand in falconer's glove, a large bird of prey on his wrist. It was taken a few days before his wedding where, instead of the usual style "stag night" he invited his close male friends to spend some time in the countryside including a bird sanctuary where it was possible to have this experience.

Chapter 27

Reality of Death

Ben was so close to me, is so close to me, it makes the reality of death—of my own death—enter within, almost as if I had stepped over the threshold with him. In a sense I too have "died"; am not what I was and cannot return to what I was.

Because my relationship to him is organic, at times I feel I am "pulled" into his experience. His experience now.

There are urgent questions: "What was it like, darling? What is it like?" as if one could ask about it in the way I would ask him about any other powerful, important experience I wanted to share, hear about.

Chapter 28

Prague Postcard

Among my papers I find the postcard Ben wrote to his much-loved Jewish grandparents[1] while he was on a visit to Prague in April 1992.

The card itself is an old one, probably dating back to the beginning of the 20th century, a tinted picture of the city from across the river Vltava, the Charles Bridge in the corner . . . and chosen, I like to imagine, quite intentionally as appropriate for these very special recipients.

The message is poignant, tenderly fanciful, written from the heart, as his Koralek grandfather had died in 1983 and his Koralek grandmother in 1989:

Dearest Granny and Pa,

This postcard is a little late, but I just wanted you both to know that I've made it to Prague and Eastern Europe. The city is beautiful and alive, and has been saved from the ravages of Nazism and the attrition of Communism.

I went to an amazing synagogue today and felt proud to be alive, with your blood coursing through my veins.

With much love and special thoughts from your loving grandson,

Ben.

---

1   Ernest and Alice Koralek with their small son had fled Vienna for London in June 1938.(The British Government were willing to accept young refugees only, so they had to leave their parents behind.) It was only after the war had ended that they learned that all their parents and many other close relatives had perished in the Holocaust. All of them had lived in many parts of the Austro-Hungarian Empire.

Chapter 29

"Geological"

which valley is this?
this ground,
this plateau,
our bedrock.
they say that some rivers
have their source
at high altitude.

—poem to his parents for Christmas 1993. The words meander
river-like across an abstract but slightly Buddhist design
painted on wood in pale blue, gold, rust, purple and black

And on the back these messages:

I tried to write a poem about my sense of "family" and "home" and this
is what I ended up with.

With all my love and geological gratitude—Ben

Dearest Ma and Pa—I feel such a strong gratitude to you both for giving
me such a generous and (rock) solid experiences of HOME and what
family is to me, it is the ground, the very earth upon which I walk. And I
feel so particularly blessed with it; thanks to you both. To try and show
you the strength of these feelings I have made this small "object" as a
more or less "permanent" [in brackets he has written "Buddhist joke"
and indeed the colors are now much faded] reminder to you both of the
gratitude I have; not just for providing a very deep sense of HOME all

these years, but for bringing me up open-minded enough to embrace the possibility of deepening that sense so that I now feel prepared to (like a river) make a journey back to my source, and in doing so make my own HOME.

And the strength of all these feelings is "geological" . . .

With all my love to you both—Ben.

Only now, re-reading these messages, and as I desperately search in all his writings for "signs," "intimations," clues perhaps pointing to the development of his outer and his inner life, moving inexorably, unbeknownst, certainly to us, toward untimely death, I understand that this "deep sense of HOME," this readiness he was feeling to make his own HOME, is more about "finding himself" than the literal aim to "settle down," although I am sure that that is partly what he meant . . .

But first and foremost he was ready—far earlier than many or most—to realize the need to "return to the source," that "turning around in the deepest seat of consciousness," the Buddhists speak of, that "metanoia," the Greeks and early Christianity tell us is absolutely essential if there is to be any evolution of the human spirit during its life within the body . . . This "turning around" which seems only to become remotely possible through some huge upheaval, some huge event, which has activated our slumber, our passivity, our inert acceptance of "things as they are" . . . in Ben's case the almost unremitting struggle to live a normal life while under frequent siege from illnesses; in my case now demanded by the immense shock of his death . . .

And he had a hard time of it, in his valiant struggle to return to the source, going against the strong stream of the acceptable norm, which he had sensed increasingly was not for him: He had dreams for the world. He was searching, had been long searching through all the demanding, rewarding, often poorly paid jobs, the different studies and disciplines he accepted to undertake, in his search to find the form which was right for him, the place where his ideas, passionate ideas and wishes that a better, richer, more complete kind of education could be made available to children . . . By the time he died his voice was beginning to be heard, his words beginning to be published in the domain where others like him express such concerns and try to find ways to bring them into being. It is possible that, had he lived, he would have made a major contribution in the educational field to a way of doing things differently and better. He had a real gift for inspiring and for enthusing others which, harnessed to the practical necessities to actually make something happen, and by working with like- minded but perhaps more experienced and practical visionaries, might well have contributed worthwhile influences—changes even—into the way we educate our children.

Chapter 30

Grief Stabs

Again it is coming in stabs—grief stabs. Suddenly. Vivid reliving of many moments—above all seeing him dead in the hospital chapel . . . Waving good-bye when we left three days earlier, not knowing it was the last time we would see him alive.

Just suddenly remembering for millionth time in any day that he is dead . . . stab, stab, stab.

Is this grief an impermanent "mood" or state such as Buddhists describe and consider as transient, teach as not to be identified with, because passing, because impermanent? Is this grief that? This sudden stabbing as I go about my daily tasks? As I climb the stairs? As I try to go to sleep at night?

It can come "out of the blue," "at the drop of a hat," from some really inconsequential remark made by another, from some sudden association, from the myriad vivid memories which are my curse and my blessing.

At one moment I genuinely experience the crucible in a positive way. At another moment I cannot understand or believe I ever did.

At one moment I truly welcome "present moment, wonderful moment" and a sort of love flows from me toward him, toward everyone and everything. At another moment that cannot happen, is meaningless.

But, when I experience myself just as an "entity," a form, and can free myself from "me" and him from "he," then the perspective is quite different . . .

Chapter 31

Grief Work

With the greatest of ease I can call to mind the many other parents we know, have known, including my own mother and father, my sister, an aunt and a grandmother, as well as a considerable number of friends all over the world, who have lost children to untimely death. Sometimes it helps to be reminded how very far from being alone I am in this terrible experience.

When we meet there is either a cautious approach, a silent embrace, a tacit agreement we may not really want to talk about it much, or at all.

Two pieces of advice stay with me from one couple.

He: "You *must* keep your spirits up."

A very old man, still loving life, distinguished in the world, but above all of the greatest integrity and goodness, I knew he meant by that no false attempts at jollying oneself along, but a turning to the creative world as he still does, to all the arts, the finest arts, to friends and good company; to go out into the world and look around "at all things lovely every hour."

He said this to me, as, bent nearly double now, he kissed my hand and set off to enjoy the exhibition of the Chinese warriors.

She: "You must let it go." "I can't," I said and she murmured her understanding . . .

But I was distressed by what she had said. *Is* it *just* a mega identification, a powerful, overwhelming "attachment" in Buddhist language? Or does grief belong in some other category?

I don't yet know.

What came to me was, *I must learn to live with it*, and then the words of a Buddhist nun told to me by a friend: "Don't *add* anything," words which really speak to me every time I remember them. That seems more like it.

No sentimental ornamentation of the experience, of the feelings about it; no self-pity. In all truth I do not yet feel guilty of either: it is as if there is absolutely no room for either, it is too awful for there to be any place for them. I can only pray that it will stay like that.

And again I experience two states simultaneously, two places in myself, or two parts of myself: the "ordinary" reaction to shock-filled reminders of Ben: his slippers under the coat stand, for example . . . Anything in any room in the house: at every turn of the stair, at any given moment: all his lovely photographs of flowers in close up, of trees, their trunks, their foliage, landscapes he loved, the engineering details on the Golden Gate bridge, art books he loved to study, postcards with tender or witty messages falling out of books he gave me for Christmas and birthdays; in the garden against an ivied wall the stone carving of a winged foolish dancing pig I gave him for a birthday present the year he and his university friends invented a daft Utopia of their own complete with a national anthem, the land of "Concordia" dedicated to EATING. Special cooking ingredients in kitchen cupboards which I used exclusively for his food; even the plastic containers and flasks I used to take soups and other nourishing meals up to him in Cambridge—any of these can suddenly plunge a little knife into the solar plexus. And then I have only to step outside the front door, go out into the neighborhood in any direction and I am retracing his first steps from infancy to the last day of his last visit . . .

And then there is this other place within me seemingly connected to another world where form and ordinary memory begin to diminish, to dissolve and I am connected to him in some quite different way *at this very moment* and I know then indeed that all is well, *all shall be well,* *manner of thing shall be well.* I feel able to "offer up" my "self" and grief. Well-being fills me. Peace. There are no satisfactory words for this state.

It is immensely valuable when the two states are seen at the same moment, and I am enabled to understand at that moment that I must no longer dwell either in the one or the other *only,* but *between the two at the same time. There lies the only "hope" of living this grief, wholly, wholesomely . . .* This insight leads me to turn more often to intentional moments of sitting quietly, a straight but not rigid spinal column, extremely still, hearing silence, hearing "the blessed silence of the dead." Maybe *this* is the true meaning of "letting it go"?

Or is this "ordinary" state of reaction to grief perhaps the most powerful of identifications or attachments ever to be experienced? The greatest of "temptations" in St. Anthony's meaning of the word?

Often when I have been sitting quietly between these two worlds I find myself murmuring the prayer which Buddhists use at the end of their sitting practice as a dedication to all beings, so that their practice does not fall into the trap of well-wishing solely for one's own ego-benefit:

> *By the power and truth of this practice*
> *May all beings have happiness and the causes*
> *of happiness.*
> *May they be free from sorrow and the causes of sorrow.*
> *May they never be separated from the sacred happiness*
> *which is sorrowless.*
> *And may all live in equanimity, without too much*
> *attachment or too much aversion,*
> *And live believing in the equality of everything that lives.*

"Happiness"? Is that the right word really? Or might it be "well-being"? Or even "joy"? Or even more daringly, "Peace"? But not of the passive, complacent, "self-calming" kind considered by G. I. Gurdjieff to be the arch-antithesis of consciousness, but rather that *"Peace of God which passeth all understanding"* of St. Paul.

And there are moments of that kind of peace and then my house is filled with Ben's atmosphere. I cannot find a better word than that to describe the sense of his presence—his voice, his laugh, his foot on the stair, at the stove, cooking rice (always far too much), talking enthusiastically—"eloquence personified" as someone put it—across the kitchen table with his father about his work, opening the front door to Jehovah's witnesses and hearing them out with charm and courtesy . . . and so on and on . . .

And I bask in that atmosphere and find a lighter step, a less heavy heart, able to go on again on this never-ending path of *"Trauerarbeit"*[1] as the Germans call it, laboring over this *"travail de deuil"*[2] as the French call it.

---

1 "grief work"

2 "mourning work"

Chapter 32

A Metaphor

A metaphor offered straight from the outside world or what is commonly called "reality":

While sitting quietly this morning, before long—for once—connecting with deep silence, suddenly the screaming, piercing sound of a chain-saw penetrated.

Of course the immediate reaction was to stop. "I can't meditate with that racket going on . . ." But following very swiftly some part of me said, That sound is like the pain of your grief frequently sawing into, cutting into you. Don't refuse it. Stay here sitting quietly with the noise and the silence. It is helping you to understand how to live between both worlds simultaneously . . .

So I stayed and continued. I did not become so accustomed to the saw noise that I no longer heard it. I was able to maintain a degree of presence between the screech of grief represented by that saw and the silence, a great silence, behind it.

Chapter 33

Of Robins and Butterflies

There is no doubt at all that immediately after Ben died, and for many months after, I was acutely aware of the natural world—more so than I had ever been before. I have since learnt that this is a common experience among the bereaved. Trees—the shifting shades of green; flowers—their colors, their amazing design; the changing sky; the moon, oh yes, the moon in all her phases.

Above all, birds and butterflies—suddenly they were everywhere and close, close by . . . settling fearlessly—robins in particular seemed positively brazen . . .

What is it that makes one so very aware of the natural world at such a time?

Is it simply the general heightened awareness which was certainly my experience for a long, long time after Ben died? An all-encompassing attention—inner and outer.

Whatever brings this about, I find it is shared by many others and beautifully described by the poet, Dannie Abse, in his exceptional book, *The Presence,* written after the sudden, totally unexpected death of his wife.

In one example he is showing his daughter a poem written by the widow of the poet, Edward Blishen about "the birds that haunted her garden," which reminds the daughter of "how one open-air day . . . soon after Joan's funeral, the dainty robin that had always ventured a hardly measured distance from Joan while she was gardening, had hopped through the open kitchen door into the house and had flown through the hall, up the stairs, into our bedroom."

Elsewhere in the book he describes how he was sitting in the garden when "a solitary white butterfly floated over the bushes near the wall and I recalled the note I had written among the aphorisms in my note book: 'Should you see a white butterfly, little solitary soul, staggering in a churchyard, rising above stone tablets, then stumbling, then rising again like one learning how to fly, have the grace to stand still for a moment.' The garden was no churchyard but I stood up till the butterfly vanished . . . "

And this reminded *me* that when I went back to Ben's grave on the day he was buried when everyone had long gone away, there was a butterfly circling the grave again and again, again and again—attracted of course by the flowers . . .

Chapter 34

A New Body

Someone reminded me that the butterfly appears independently, so to speak, of the caterpillar and the chrysalis ...

The cocoon completely "disappears," crumbles? Liquidates? It is no more.

The butterfly is a new body ...

And yet ... could it appear without the caterpillar and the chrysalis? Another example of a "sea change," an "exchange of substances" (in the words of G. I. Gurdjieff)?

In any case, this lovely image of something new and beautiful and winged somehow touched me and also reminded me that according to Plato, the butterfly represents the soul.

Chapter 35

Ben's Words

A birthday card falls out of a book: "Happy Birthday Mum, our culture-vulture! No! Our culture-*condor*!"

"Mum, I sometimes think the words I use most to you are either: 'Thanks, Mum' or 'Sorry, Mum!'"

His sister Lucy reminds me how, when he felt things were getting tense, negative in the family circle, he would say with a wonderful lightly serious intonation: "*Steady!*"

I am so grateful for this reminder and find myself hearing it often now when the dark side makes itself felt.

Chapter 36

Cantus Firmus

Pin your faith on the cantus firmus.[1]

There is nothing to save, now all is lost
But a tiny core in the stillness of the heart,
Like the eye of a violet.[2]

During his last, cruel illness, Michael Mayne, the courageous, life-loving and perceptive Dean Emeritus of Westminster, somehow managed to write *The Enduring Melody*, an immensely generous and inspiring meditation on his rich life and approaching death.

The title is his translation of the musical term, *"cantus firmus"* or "ground bass," which he has used as a perfect metaphor for the firm ground we all need to stand upon while the force of life flows, surges, overwhelms us with its immense gamut, which includes every kind of joy and rejoicing, every degree of suffering. Perfect metaphor if we equate all the melody, counterpoint, harmonies that weave around the *cantus firmus* in music—in Bach for example—with that immense gamut . . .

But . . . if I am honest I so easily lose contact with that firm ground . . .

But . . . I am called, now more than ever since Ben's death, to return

---

1 Dietrich Bonhoeffer, the heroically outspoken German pastor in a letter written in prison to a close friend just before he was executed by the Nazis and quoted by Michael Mayne in *The Enduring Melody*.

2 D. H. Lawrence quoted by Michael Mayne in *The Enduring Melody*.

to that contact. What calls? Who calls? If I say I don't know I am not being honest; if I say I *do* know I am also not being honest. The word "mystery" so easily bandied about really comes into its own here.

I *do* know now that the contact is related to the stillness which D. H. Lawrence describes in such simple language in his poem written about some great loss of his own. Stillness—finding room for it daily—becomes more and more necessary, crucial, if I am to make this contact once more. Stillness first of the body, which can lead to thoughts and feelings becoming more subdued—their impermanence now seen, having less power over me. Stillness, leading to silence: first my own relative silence, then I hear absolute silence . . . Counted in ordinary time measures these moments are brief, but their impact, their impression does indeed impress itself in me, leave an inward mark upon me.

Near the end of his wonderful book, Michael Mayne puts into words exactly what I feel Ben was moving toward understanding in his last year . . .

"To die with gratitude for all that has been, without resentment for what you are going through, and with openness toward the future, is the greatest gift we can leave those who love us and who are left behind."

And expressing this in another way a friend wrote to us when Ben died:

> Surely what matters is that Ben lived fully, that there was love in his life, given and received, as he learned and grew through his struggles, as must all of those who were close to him.

I have written elsewhere in this book of Ben's lifelong sense of gratitude—he had not time to say anything about it at the end, but I think and feel that it was an ingredient—a large one—of his own particular *cantus firmus*.

Chapter 37

Meditation on Psalm 121

I will lift up mine eyes unto the hills:
From whence cometh my help.
My help cometh even from the Lord: who hath made
heaven and earth.
He will not suffer thy foot to be moved: and he that
keepeth thee will not sleep.
Behold, he that keepeth Israel: shall neither slumber
nor sleep.
The Lord himself is thy keeper: the Lord is thy defense
upon thy right hand.
So that the sun shall not burn thee by day, neither
the moon by night.
The Lord shall preserve thee from all evil: yea, it is even
he that shall preserve thy soul.
The Lord shall preserve thy going out and thy coming in:
from this day forth for evermore.

—Psalm 121 in The Book of Common Prayer

We sang this psalm at Ben's funeral.

I have always loved it ever since the days we sang it, often, at school and the words had been in me once more during the last year or so of Ben's life. But now they seem to be taking on a deeper meaning. "The Lord" for me had come to represent the experiences I was receiving more often than ever before throughout my life of a Goodness, a

Benevolence which seemed to descend upon me every time I felt myself to be "on the floor" with anxiety, despair and anguish over Ben's frequent suffering...

I began to understand that at those moments I had the choice of either going down and down into subjective depths of misery and helplessness, or of "looking upwards" and "offering up" the helplessness in an act of faith—offering it to I knew not what, yet... there was an instinctive feeling or sense that that was the only thing I could "do"...

It seemed the absolutely right psalm to sing at the funeral—an act of faith, but also as if we were talking to Ben, assuring him that he was cared for by our great love but above all, or at least also, by this Goodness, this Benevolence, this Love... which would not *suffer his foot to be moved*, would not let him *stumble*, would not let him be *burned* either by the sun or the moon; would watch over his *coming and going* and all because, unlike us, *the Lord God of Israel neither slumbers nor sleeps*, this Lord God, this Goodness, this Benevolence, this Love is the ultimate Awakened One. And yet, as I write this, I seem to know that there is within me such a One and that One accompanies Ben here, now, always ...

When I decided to reflect further on this psalm I looked for other versions:

Psalm 121 A Song of degrees

I will lift up mine eyes unto the hills
From whence cometh my help.
My help cometh from the Lord, which made heaven
    and earth.
He will not suffer thy foot to be moved; he that keepeth
    thee will not slumber.
Behold, he that keepeth Israel shall neither slumber
    nor sleep.
The Lord is thy keeper: the Lord is thy shade upon
    thy right hand.
The sun shall not smite thee by day, nor the moon
    by night.

The Lord shall preserve thee from all evil: he shall
preserve thy soul.
The Lord shall preserve thy going out and thy coming
in from this time forth, and even forevermore.

—King James translation

Psalm 121 The guardian of Israel

Song of Ascents
I lift up my eyes to the mountains;
Where is my help come from?
My help comes from Yahweh
Who made heaven and earth.
May he save your foot from stumbling;
May he, your guardian, not fall asleep!
You see—he neither sleeps nor slumbers,
The guardian of Israel.
Yahweh is your guardian, your shade,
Yahweh, at your right hand.
By day the sun will not strike you,
Nor the moon by night.
Yahweh guards you from all harm
Yahweh guards your life,
Yahweh guards your comings and goings,
Henceforth and forever.

—New Jerusalem Bible[1]

The description of this psalm—both in the King James version of the
Bible and the New Jerusalem Bible—as "A song of degrees," "A song of

---

1 The question mark after "from whence cometh my help" only appears in this translation, but would seem to make very good sense, turning the next line into a response:
"my help cometh even from the Lord..."

Ascents" touched me deeply, conveying this image of looking upwards with faith to this Goodness which cares for us.

Further studies brought me to the *Nine Talmudic Readings*—lectures given by the eminent Jewish scholar and philosopher, the late Emmanuel Levinas. There I discovered that he had a radical view of the meaning of "the Lord God of Israel" where he seems to imply that "Israel" could be taken to signify the entire human community.[1]

But further reflection brought me back to remembering I had found more than one source suggesting that the inner meaning of YHWH is sometimes interpreted in mystical, esoteric Judaism as "I AM"—the ultimate affirmation of presence, a presence which by definition "neither slumbers nor sleeps."

And from there I returned to the opening words of the great Jewish prayer, the Shema, whose first line is usually translated as: "Hear, O Israel, the Lord thy God is one," but I found in a scholarly study that in fact that "one" might be "oneness" (or even, even more interestingly, perhaps added to make sense where once the words would have petered out into silence in front of the unspeakable, the ineffable, the unknowable); that the first part of the word "Israel" in Hebrew "ish" (which means "being" or "a being") could incline toward the meaning of a being who tries to ascend toward "God," toward "I AM" . . . (the "el" being one Hebrew word for one level of meaning of "God" and the "ra" of "Is-ra-el" indicates movement).

I lean on this psalm, the understanding within it, the conviction within it, that there is this help—above me.

---

1 *Judaism and Revolution*

Chapter 38

"Marvelous"

Nearly two years after Ben died, a bright spring day, returning from a satisfying shopping spree before going to visit friends in California, approaching our front door I hear myself say out loud, wholeheartedly, happily, "*Mar*velous!"

And laugh to hear that it sounded just the way Ben used to say that—with a lovely breathy joyful sound: "*Mar*-velous!"

And wept.

Chapter 39

Now Dreams Come

I longed for dreams soon after he died. Dreams of meeting him, but they never came.

But now they come, powerfully and painfully.

In one he is a baby in a cot. He is ill. I am fussing endlessly with the bedclothes, re-arranging them this way and that. The room is already darkened with blinds pulled down, but I go to them again and again to fiddle with them. He is standing up in the cot—a baby—in a long gown. I hold him, hold him so tightly it is as if we melt into one another. It is a sweet feeling.

But I wake up very sad. The dream is no comfort. Somehow earlier I thought dreams would be.

In another one, he is the grown good-looking man he was until he died, standing at a slight distance on the threshold of a doorway.

His sister, Lucy, is there too just behind me.

"I don't want to be separated from you, Mum," he is saying. "I don't want to be separated from you either, Luce . . . "

I go to him and hold him again so tightly we seem to become almost one. There is such a feeling of such love.

"We won't be separated, darling," I say to him. "Because we are all three made from the same cells . . . "

Again, this dream hurts.

Chapter 40

Californian Postscript

May 2008

"You were wide open . . . " said one of the friends I had visited in San Francisco, as we talked over my days there . . .

Certainly a lot of powerful experiences came to me there . . .

Dreams[1]

I

How I have longed for them and had so very few, but now they came thick and fast: very painful, flinging me out of bed in the very early morning out into the lovely garden where I was staying:
I am nursing a sick baby . . . there is a crib . . . I am endlessly arranging and re-arranging the bedding for the baby's maximum comfort. The blinds are down, the room is rather dark. The baby is wearing a long nightgown . . . I keep pressing the baby to my heart . . . the baby feels "thin" like a paper doll, not real full flesh and plumpness . . .

II

Ben is there, grown and looking just like he did toward the end of his life . . . dressed in grey. He is moving toward a doorway. I am near him, behind him, and Lucy is near me, behind me . . . "I can't come home for two or three months," he is saying. I hug him and implore

---

1 Astonished to find that I had already recorded both these dreams on 14 April, about ten days before I left for California (see Now Dreams Come) but in slightly different forms.

him, "But I can look after you! I know how to look after you . . . !" But he just keeps saying, "I can't come home, Mum, not for two or three months . . . " And then he says something to both Lucy and me, something generous, loving, caring, but I can no longer remember the actual words but there remains some sense of a farewell in them . . . and he goes toward that door . . . and I wake up and that's when I leap up and rush into the peaceful early morning flower-filled sanctuary . . .

Chapter 41

Tonglen[1]

One evening while I was in California, when my hostess was out, I tried Tonglen.

All I heard myself say was, "the grief is colossal," and sensed that my "meditation" for Tonglen was not yet strong enough.

But one morning early, in that quiet house, I tried again. I "saw" "Jenny" facing me and was able to some degree to "draw off" her suffering.

And I don't really think that at this level of trying it matters much that the first words that came to me were from Christ: *Before Abraham was I AM.*

And then I heard, "Mum, Mum"; said "Ben, Ben, I am with you."

"We're in this together, Mum."

Saw "Jenny" belongs to the solidity of *form* and *Before Abraham was, I AM* to *formlessness* where Ben and I meet and where he is not Ben form and I am not Jenny form, and that this applies to us all. We get trapped in form, ego, persona, *petite personne,* but the other, the I AM is free, molecular, atomic, flowing into a great "sea." Formless Ben dwells there and I meet him there.

Can this insight be brought to bear on how we relate to one another here in our "planetary bodies"?

I felt this was a very important moment.

---

1 See for example in *The Tibetan Book of Living and Dying* by Sogyal Rinpoche and in other contemporary and, of course, much older Tibetan Buddhist texts.

"I am with you"; he with me; me with him—but "Ben," "Mum" is secondary to this other formless, atomic "meltdown."

Already these words are a translation. The impression of what happened and what is happening is not this formulation but prajna, gnosis, or in the words of Henri Tracol, *la primauté de l'expérience*, "the immediacy of the experience."

Not long before I left for California I was so troubled in myself about this never-ending grief and my attitudes to it that I "decided" I needed counseling . . .

I spent a long evening trawling the internet for local therapists, offering help with all manner of "issues"; There were dozens of them. How on earth could I know which one might be right for me; good at their job?

And suddenly it came to me that this was not the help I was really looking for; that I needed to be active in my search for understanding. An outpouring onto someone else, a sort of expectation that someone else would take the burdensome experience off me, suddenly seemed a very passive approach and that I needed one that was not so much psychological as spiritual. "There must be something like that," I muttered, "in Buddhism, say?" And a dim memory came to me of a practice I had even learned long ago at a Tibetan Buddhist center . . .

Yes. *Tonglen*, or the practice of "giving and receiving," also sometimes described as "The Holy Secret." How could I have forgotten that I had not only learned it, but had practiced it many times for Ben . . . ? Not for the first time I found myself wondering why, why, why I forget so easily what I have "known" and let alone what I have at times "understood."

I do not believe that sacred practices should be described as if they were recipes. And also each of us needs to find the help which is "right" for them.

But the hint is in the words "giving and receiving."

Chapter 42

"My Stroke of Insight"

I had not expected to be so profoundly affected by watching, while in California, this twenty minute film online—a talk given by Jill Bolte Taylor on her extraordinary experiences observing herself having a stroke.

She was able to watch the division in her brain—the separation—between a kind of blissful dissolution, melting impression, experience of her atom-ness, her particle-ness and the joy of that, the freedom of that, while at the same time seeing the mind which goes with form acting reasonably—working out how to call for help, describing the process she was going through. It really seemed that she was witnessing her two worlds, her two natures, the higher and the lower simultaneously, something I and many others strive for almost daily—to be present to them both at the same time and, as she so passionately acknowledged, understanding that both are needed.

But she wept as she described losing the contact with the molecular, melted, formless part of herself and the return, painful, but at that moment still possible, and necessary if she were to survive, to the world of form.

I had not expected to have to leave the room and withdraw and weep with joy and relief: so this must have been what Ben experienced—that joyous dissolving . . . and I was reminded of his description of sensing he was happily slipping away after losing a great deal of blood . . . and of other descriptions I have come across of near death experiences where the person always seems to have been sad to "have to come back" . . .

This vivid, totally convincing account of a miraculous "stroke of insight" stays with me as a rare (in our time) "proof" of ancient descriptions of the process of leaving the physical body and has brought a kind of "scientific" comfort . . . It is *all right* . . .

Chapter 43

Ben's Other Side

Perhaps I have made Ben sound to have been a man without failings.

Of course this is not so, and, feeling that it would not be right to ex-
clude any mention of them, I was reminded of a passage in Gurdjieff's
book, *Life is Real, Only Then, When "I AM,"* where he tells of an ancient custom that, living in an age where any mention or thought of
death is largely taboo, seems shocking. Long, long ago, when someone
died those who had known him gathered together at a "Remembering
Feast." There they would recall only his bad qualities and would eat only
the food which had been prepared in advance by the one who had died
(which for me signifies that he understood and welcomed the reasons
for the gathering; welcomed the fact that his death could be of positive
help to others).

> *And this they did daily for three days . . . After this pe-*
> *culiar three-day procedure all those who had taken part*
> *gathered daily for seven days . . . All present sat or kneeled*
> *quietly and began to give themselves up to the contempla-*
> *tion of the inevitability of their own death . . .*

And they would pray for help to keep death always before their eyes.

Gurdjieff concludes by saying:
> *I will leave it to each one of you to decide for himself what*
> *advantage there might be if such a "savage" custom could*
> *be established again.*

Well, all who knew Ben would agree wryly, even bitterly perhaps, that he was hopeless with money . . . certainly not in any way dishonest, just very extravagant, very generous, but seemingly unable to keep a realistic, practical eye on expenditure or cut his coat according to his cloth. (I should add that thanks to Vicky, he was beginning to get better at doing so.)

He was also exceedingly romantic, which could lead to enchantingly imaginative acts of tenderness, but also to the hurt of unrealistic and therefore unsustainable relationships.

Chapter 44

What Can I Lean Into?

In all the honesty I can muster is there anything I can lean into when I hit the floor?

Is there ever any real help, comfort in any wisdom, either spoken to me, or among the wide-ranging sacred texts I have ransacked over the past two years?

I now have the picture of courageous Jill Bolte Taylor, observing herself moving between the two worlds we undoubtedly inhabit even if mostly unbeknownst to us . . .

I have the words sent me about the man, *who, when he departs this world,* all in act *having done what there is to be done, need not wonder what will become of him, nor where he is going, but will inevitably find the bull's eye and passing through the sun door enter the empyrean beyond the* murity *of the sky.*

I have the words from the Upanishad, *Through the heart flows a food finer than the food that nourishes the body.*

I have *In my father's house are many mansions.*

I have *Before Abraham was, I AM.* These are the words I perhaps to return to most often. Their meaning seems to grow in me: if I understand them rightly: the horizontal of ordinary time represented in *before Abraham was,* the vertical of outside time in those two small strong words, *I AM.*

When I murmur them to myself at times of utmost darkness I do

seem to understand that this "I AM" is not me, it goes beyond and behind me and in that sense is immortal; and therefore likewise Ben's I
AMness is too.

And then there is the immense help of the gentle words of Sri Anirvan in his piece Life-Death[1] (the complete text worthy of repeated
study and attempts to put into practice):

> ... the moment of physical death or of passage to a lighter
> density, is a moment of transubstantiation, a function of
> the spirit informed by sensation... One enters a new field
> of forces. Does one know what is going to happen when
> arriving on earth? Why would it not be the same thing
> after death? There may be as many solutions in death as
> there are in life. One follows, it is certain, a road opened
> by an exact Law.

I have the words of a friend, words which can only have come from his
own experience:

> Oh Jenny, what suffering for you both and for Ben's wife
> and child. I do feel that grief has to be respected absolute-
> ly and lived, until, in its own time, it becomes less central,
> less burning. The Good Lord does seem to have made us
> so that we can withstand the bitterest events and know
> that we can and must go on living and contributing. The
> place of grief shifts from the center of the chest to some
> eternal inner corner, always there but no longer requiring
> the same attention, no longer stopping the manifestation
> of one's own bright energy. Maybe that energy will have a
> trace always of the color of the person who died, but that
> is not a bad thing, the color is beautiful.

All, when I am able to remember them, bring real help.

---

1 In *To Live Within*, Sri Anirvan and Lizelle Reymond, Morning Light Press, 2007.

But above all, when I am able to remember them, it is Ben's own words which are the most healing balm, written to comfort me on the death of Henri Tracol's widow:

> *I am sure that people of such quality do not really "go" anywhere—they just "change" their form. I am sure she has become part of you . . .*

And "yes" I see that it is indeed so: the ones truly, fully loved are always part of us, can "be" with us at any moment—and one's child more than any: part of me long before birth; part of me after death for the remainder of my days and beyond . . .

Such love, such gratitude, such a blessing . . . . Ben . . .

These moments of heightened awareness, deeper understanding, clearer vision, when they come, at their purest come from my son, my child . . . through whom, through this form, this human form of a special, sun and star-filled being came, and still now comes, my experience of great love, unconditional love, devotion . . . this "light" offered at this colossal cost of his death . . . and now . . . for what? I owe it to him—or to what he represents now formless, to "go forward" in the words of Hermann Hesse; to allow this feeling of being undone, of not knowing, of being completely broken, to become a transforming substance, a-working on me not just for myself but for the sake of all "sentient beings," so that, inspired by Ben's example, these words of Gurdjieff's may now really and deeply penetrate my thought, my heart and my marrowbone:

> *I am thou,*
> *Thou art I,*
> *He is ours,*
> *So all may be for our neighbor.[1]*

---

1 Meetings with Remarkable Men (Penguin, 1991).

I think Ben was a shooting star.

—A childhood friend

I am sure that Ben's goodness and sweetness will see him raised to something of which we have no knowledge.

—in a letter from a friend, July 2006

Birth and death cannot be applied to reality.

—Thich Nhat Hanh, 1987

. . . your sorrow is for nothing. The wise grieve neither for
the living nor for the dead.
Nor I, nor thou, ever was not, nor ever will not be.
All that doth live, lives always.
To man's frame as there come infancy and youth
and age,
So come there raisings-up and layings-down
Of other life-abodes
Which the wise know, and fear not.
The unreal has no being.
That which is real can never cease to be . . .

—The Bhagavad Gita Book II, c.500 BCE

Acknowledgements

Page 17
From *The Complete Poems* by C Day Lewis published by Sinclair-Stevenson (1992) Copyright © 1992 in this edition The Estate of C Day Lewis. Reprinted by permission of The Random House Group Ltd.

Pages 48–9; also page 82
From *A Voice at the Borders of Silence: An Intimate Look at the Gurdjieff Work, Zen Buddhism and Art* by William Segal, with Marielle Bancou-Segal. Copyright © 2003 Marielle Bancou-Segal. Reprinted by permission of The Overlook Press, New York, NY. All rights reserved. www.overlook-press.com

Page 56
The Poetics of Space, Gaston Bachelard, Beacon Press, Boston,1994.

Page 107
From *Luminous Emptiness* by Francesca Fremantle, Copyright 2001, by Francesca Fremantle. Reprinted by arrangement with Shambhala Publications Inc., Boston, MA. www.shambhala.com

Page 134–5
The Presence, by Dannie Abse, Hutchinson, London 2007. Reprinted by kind permission of the author.

Page 138
Taken from *The Enduring Melody*, by Michael Mayne, published and copyright © 2006 by Darton Longman and Todd Ltd. London and used by permission of the publishers.